THE HRT
SOLUTION

THE HRT SOLUTION

*A comprehensive, personalized program
of natural hormone replacement to relieve
menopausal symptoms and restore vitality,
sexuality, and health . . . for life*

Second Edition

MARLA AHLGRIMM, R.PH.
and JOHN M. KELLS
with
CHRISTINE MACGENN RODGERSON

AVERY
a member of Penguin Group (USA) Inc.
New York
2003

Every effort has been made to ensure that the information contained in this book is complete and accurate. However, neither the publisher nor the authors are engaged in rendering professional advice or services to the individual reader. The ideas, procedures, and suggestions contained in this book are not intended as a substitute for consulting with your physician. All matters regarding health require medical supervision. Neither the authors nor the publisher shall be liable or responsible for any loss, injury, or damage allegedly arising from any information or suggestion in this book. The opinions expressed in this book represent the personal views of the authors and not of the publisher.

Most Avery books are available at special quantity discounts for bulk purchase for sales promotions, premiums, fund-raising, and educational needs. Special books or book excerpts also can be created to fit specific needs. For details, write Penguin Group (USA) Inc. Special Markets, 375 Hudson Street, New York, NY 10014.

a member of
Penguin Group (USA) Inc.
375 Hudson Street
New York, NY 10014
www.penguin.com

Library of Congress Cataloging-in-Publication Data

Ahlgrimm, Marla.
HRT Solution : a comprehensive, personalized program of natural hormone replacement to relieve menopausal symptoms and restore vitality, sexuality, and health . . . for life / Marla Ahlgrimm and John M. Kells ; with Christine Macgenn Rodgerson.
p. cm.
Includes bibliographical references and index.
ISBN 1-58333-176-X
1. Menopause–Hormone therapy—Popular works.   2. Menopause—Alternative treatment—Popular works.   I. Kells, John M.   II. Macgenn, Christine.   III. Title.
RG186.A35   2003   2003048106
618.1'75061—dc21

Printed in the United States of America
5   7   9   10   8   6

Book design by Tanya Maiboroda

To every woman who has ever been told by her doctor,
"It's all in your head."

Acknowledgments

I am deeply thankful to those who made this book come to life. First and foremost, to the tens of thousands of women and caring professionals across the country who have shared our sense of excitement and discovery and who made it possible for us to begin to unravel the mysteries of hormones. To Christine Macgenn Rodgerson, the gifted writer who stayed inspired, stayed the course, and kept the creative process alive, my sincere gratitude. To Treacy Colbert for her creative insight, her editorial review and skill, and her unwavering commitment to our mission, my heartfelt thanks. I am also grateful to my dedicated and professional staff at Madison Pharmacy Associates, especially Debra Short for her loyalty and support. Special thanks go to Sue Taggart for her belief in this project and her efforts to help us get our message out.

To Renee Dorazio, R.N., whose tireless support, energy, encouragement, and commitment have made much of this work possible, I am deeply appreciative.

—MARLA AHLGRIMM

My gratitude to Christine Macgenn Rodgerson, whose unique writing talent and creativity molded the thoughts and ideas of this book into a meaningful and understandable story. Christine's ability to listen to and then interpret and organize complicated concepts presented from vastly different points of view were the foundation of this project.

In order to change the way medicine is practiced, one needs the guidance of an expert clinician like Dr. Charles Dollbaum, who is an objective scientist and practicing clinical oncologist. He provided much of the medical and technical guidance for this material. My appreciation to the staff of Aeron LifeCycles Clinical Laboratory, whose scientific expertise meets the daily challenges and demands of an ever-increasing volume of testing with excellence and accuracy. My particular thanks to Gail Duwe for all of her editorial suggestions and careful review of this book. Thanks to Dr. Adeline Hackett for her lifelong commitment to the study of breast cancer and for her invaluable review of and input into the manuscript. Thanks to Judy Lane, a nurse practitioner dedicated to women's health issues, for her contributions. Also, my gratitude goes to Treacy Colbert for her skillful editorial review and valuable contributions. And to Shannon Whitney for her commitment to our mission and her insightful review of the manuscript.

Thanks to my wife Beby, a woman empowered to change the medical establishment, for her continued and active involvement in the tone and direction of this book.

—JOHN M. KELLS

The authors would also like to express their gratitude to John Duff, Eileen Bertelli, Kristen Jennings, Amy Tecklenburg, and the staff at Avery/Penguin Group (USA) Inc. for their enthusiasm, support, and guidance and for making our vision of this book a reality.

Contents

What About the Breast Cancer Risk?
Play It Again—The Estrogen-Progesterone Pas de Deux
Evaluating the Data on HRT and Cancer

6. CHANGING THE STATUS QUO

Out with the Old, in with the New
Understanding Replacement Hormones
Lock and Key
A Little Goes a Long Way

7. HOW DO I KNOW IF HRT IS RIGHT FOR ME?

Old, Outmoded Standards Have to Go
Your Spitting Image: Saliva Testing
Why Haven't I Heard About Saliva Testing?
Your Individual Hormonal Profile
Saliva Testing and Your Response to HRT

8. PHARMACY FOR THE TWENTY-FIRST CENTURY

Tablets, Patches, Creams, and More
Suppositories
Orals: Capsules and Tablets
Transdermals
Symptoms as a Hormonal Barometer

9. PROTECTION FOR YOUR BONES

Important Pieces of the Picture
Bone Mineral Density Tests
Bone-Resorption Testing: An Investment Counselor
for Your Bones

EPILOGUE: THE FUTURE OF HRT

Preface to the Second Edition

Hormone replacement therapy (HRT) is the practice of taking supplemental hormones to make up for those your body is no longer producing. These replacement hormones are prescribed to relieve symptoms of premenstrual syndrome, perimenopause, and menopause—all of the hormonal transitions of a woman's life. They can be prescribed for fertility problems or to help prevent bone loss and protect against other chronic degenerative diseases often associated with aging.

The conventional form of HRT consists of one-size-fits-all doses of synthetic or animal-derived hormones. Synthetic and animal-derived hormones, while the most studied, are not the same as the hormones your body makes. They perform differently in the body and can cause troublesome side effects.

We originally wrote *The HRT Solution* because we believed that this conventional, cookie-cutter form of HRT was an outmoded, ineffective, and even potentially harmful way to prescribe hormones. We still do. We wanted women to know then that they had another choice, and we want them to know it now. It is more important than ever for women to know that one-size-fits-all HRT is not all there is. Today women can choose individualized, natural hormone replacement—a higher form of health care. Natural hormones, which are derived from plants, are identical to human hormones. In fact, once they are absorbed into your body, natural hormones are indistinguishable from your own. There couldn't be a better time for the release of this new edition of *The HRT Solution*.

When we released the first edition of this book in 1999, HRT was one of the hottest topics of debate among scientists, researchers, physicians, and pharmacists. Research was telling us that there was a brave new world of longevity and fitness ahead and that our hormones could very well be the keys. We were being told that hormone replacement could reverse the aging process, improve our quality of life, protect us from disease, and increase our life span. Scientific studies were showing that taking replacement hormones could prevent bone loss in perimenopausal, menopausal, and postmenopausal women and decrease their risk of heart disease. Women who took HRT were also shown to be at lower risk for colon cancer and Alzheimer's disease. Tooth decay was decreased by HRT. Studies were even demonstrating that people who used HRT lived longer than those who did not. It was an exciting time in women's health and hormone care.

Among all the sensational headlines, however, there were some conflicting reports. Some studies were indicating that a more cautionary approach to hormone replacement might be in order. Some researchers found that conventional HRT could increase a woman's risk of developing endometrial or ovarian cancer or increase her breast cancer risk. But in spite of these reports, the good news seemed to outweigh the bad, and millions of women were taking standardized, one-size-fits-all doses of synthetic and animal-derived HRT. Even women without menopausal symptoms were taking them in the hope that they would offer some protection against many of the ravages of aging. The most popular and widely used replacement hormones were the Premarin family of products manufactured by Wyeth-Ayerst Laboratories, one of the largest pharmaceutical companies in the world. Prescribed in one-size-fits-all doses, these hormone products were considered the gold standard in hormone replacement.

Then, in the spring of 2000, the Heart and Estrogen/Progestin Hormone Replacement Study (HERS) found that, among postmenopausal women who already had heart disease, conventional HRT increased the risk of having a heart attack, stroke, or embolism within the first year of use. This was not good news. Something that was supposed to prevent heart disease now appeared to make it worse. However, the women of the HERS trial who took HRT for three to five years appeared to have a decreased risk. Because of this, study participants were asked to continue the trial to determine whether or not the decreased risk persisted after five years. HERS II went on until the spring of 2002, when findings showed that the decreased risk did not continue in years six through eight.

Right on the heels of the HERS II results, in the summer of 2002, the Women's Health Initiative (WHI), a major multiphase hormone study investigating the safety and effectiveness of two of the most popular forms of conventional HRT—Premarin and Prempro—brought one of its three trials to a screeching halt. The WHI was government-funded and sponsored by the National Institutes of Health (NIH). There had never before been a hormone study of its magnitude. The study's report of an increased risk of heart disease, breast cancer, and blood clots among the women taking Prempro sent a shock wave through the scientific and medical communities and made headlines around the world.

The news sent scores of women racing to their medicine cabinets to throw out their replacement hormones. Doctors' offices were deluged with calls from concerned women, many demanding to be taken off HRT immediately. Many of these women had suffered debilitating symptoms during menopause, symptoms that were difficult if not impossible to relieve without the aid of HRT. The thought of returning to sleepless nights, the embarrassment and discomfort of unbearable hot flashes, mood swings that made them feel like they were on an emotional roller coaster, and painful sex due to vaginal dryness seemed daunting at best. But the news was frightening. No one wanted to be taking medication that they believed to be helping them only to find out that it might be doing them harm.

Regrettably, many doctors were as taken aback by the WHI results as everyone else. They were going through their patient lists and calling all of the women who were taking Prempro and cautioning them to stop. Over 600,000 women—nearly a third of those taking it—stopped taking Prempro immediately. More than 15 percent of the women taking Premarin did the same. Within weeks, many of these women were once again experiencing their symptoms and a sudden and steep decline in their quality of life. Rivers of sweat in the middle of the night not only are uncomfortable and disconcerting but also rob a woman of a good night's sleep. Lack of sleep, anxiety, depression, fatigue, and brain fog can make a woman's life miserable. Within months, many of the women who had stopped HRT decided to start taking it again, even though they were frightened. Many of them didn't know what else to do. This may not have been necessary. There is another choice. Natural, individualized hormone replacement can relieve symptoms without the side effects that come with conventional HRT.

The arm of the WHI study that was so abruptly ended was designed to evaluate the long-term health effects of only *one* form of *conventional* HRT—Prempro—a combination of conjugated estrogens, derived from the urine of pregnant mares, and medroxyprogesterone acetate, a synthetic progestin. After five years, the study found that Prempro increased rather than decreased a woman's risk of heart disease, stroke, blood clots, and breast cancer. Other forms of hormone replacement were not tested. In addition, all of the women in the study were given exactly the same pill. It was one-size-fits-all HRT. One-size-fits-all hormone replacement is about as sensible for women as one-size-fits-all shoes.

Imagine this for a moment: The government has decided to fund a study to determine the safety of shoes. Study participants are all given a pair of size 6 shoes to wear. Women who are forced to wear shoes that don't fit begin complaining, and as the study progresses complaints of discomfort increase. The complaints are well founded. Many women are suffering from foot problems. Just think of how the headlines might read two years into the study: *Shoes Are Not Safe! Women Urged to Stop Wearing Shoes! Shoes Cause Blisters, Arch Deformities, and Crippled Toes!*

Shoes are not unsafe. But shoes that do not fit do present problems. HRT that doesn't fit also creates problems. Women don't all wear the same size shoes, and they don't all have the same hormone requirements. Hormone dosages must be individualized.

The findings of the Women's Health Initiative study actually confirm our belief that hormone replacement therapy is neither as simple as one-size-fits-all nor as benign as was once believed. Hormone replacement therapy should be administered in the same way insulin is—according to need. Not all women need hormone replacement. Insulin is never prescribed simply because a woman craves sweets or has other symptoms of blood-sugar problems. She is tested first to determine if her body is producing enough insulin. Once she is given a prescription, she is monitored carefully to make sure her insulin level stays within the physiologic range that is right for her, neither too high nor too low. The proper administration of insulin improves the quality of life for millions of people every year. Individualized natural hormone replacement can do the same.

Symptoms are one indication that hormone levels may be low. However, symptoms alone cannot determine whether you need hormone replacement. Symptoms can be caused by other factors. Decades of research and experience in women's health and hormones have taught us that hormone replacement should be prescribed only after a woman's hormone levels have been tested to determine precisely what is happening in her body hormonally. She should be given a replacement hormone only if her level of that hormone has declined, and it should be prescribed only in the lowest amount necessary to restore her levels. And she should be monitored during her therapy to evaluate how her body is responding.

When applied properly, hormone replacement has many benefits— symptomatic relief of menopausal symptoms and a decreased risk of osteoporosis, colon cancer, tooth decay, and even Alzheimer's disease are among them. Whether you are thirty-something, forty-something, fifty-something, or beyond, some of the most pressing health concerns you have may be hormone related. We believe that individualized, natural hormone replacement can be used for the short term to manage symptoms of menopause and over the long term to prevent chronic degenerative diseases.

Historically, scientists, researchers, and physicians have interpreted the results of medical studies. Now, however, because of the rising public demand for information regarding all areas of health and safety, journalists and news anchors report on studies as soon as they are released. Findings are often splashed across the front page or featured on the evening news before they have been fully interpreted and certainly well before they have actually been deemed to be factual. In their race to get a big story out first, media outlets often report scientific studies only partially, as evidenced by the media blitz surrounding the WHI results. This rapid-fire approach to reporting scientific findings isn't in anyone's best interest.

We are living in the age of information. Technology is giving us faster and faster access to more and more information all the time. But we must use discretion in how we respond to that information. Much analysis has been given to the findings of the HERS and HERS II trials. A number of inconsistencies have been revealed. Questions have been raised concerning the participants' use of statins in the original trial. Statins are cholesterol-reducing drugs that can decrease the risk of heart disease. Upon closer examination of the trial results, some researchers questioned whether the increase in cardiovascular events was real or appeared to be significant because of a *decrease* in events in the placebo group due to statin use. Also of note, only 45 percent of the women taking HRT were still using it as prescribed by year six of HERS II. It is difficult to reach reliable conclusions when there are such dramatic changes in the numbers of participants in a study.

The reporting on the WHI study was incomplete at best. The real story of the WHI had more to do with the fact that a drug—Prempro—that was approved by the FDA for the prevention of heart disease was found, in fact, to increase a woman's risk. Because of this startling evidence, there was a feeding frenzy in the media, and the entire study became bad news. You may be surprised to know that the increased risks found in the WHI were actually *slight* increased risks for women with existing heart disease. And that the study was multiphased and also reported significant good news: Hormone replacement provided a 37 percent reduction in colorectal cancer, a 33 percent decrease in hip fractures, and a 24 percent decrease in fractures in other bones.

Not long after the WHI released its findings regarding Prempro and heart disease, reports came from the WHI Memory Study (WHIMS) regarding Prempro use and cognition in women. WHIMS was a substudy within the WHI designed to assess the effects of Premarin and Prempro on memory and other cognitive functions: attention, concentration, language, abstract reasoning, and calculation. WHIMS was investigating whether the use of these hormone replacement products lowered a woman's risk of normal cognitive decline (decrease in memory and other thinking abilities), mild cognitive impairment or MCI (a noteworthy decrease in at least one cognitive skill), and dementia (a significant decline in multiple cognitive capabilities that interferes with normal daily functions and that is not the result of other medical conditions. Because the Prempro arm of the WHI was ended early, the WHIMS data on Prempro and cognition became available sooner than anticipated.

WHIMS found that Prempro use did not protect women from normal cognitive decline. In fact, women who were taking the combination drug actually performed more poorly on cognitive tests than the women on a placebo. In addition, Prempro use was found to increase the risk of dementia. Women taking Prempro were twice as likely as women who weren't to develop dementia over the course of the study. Again, the results were startling. A drug that was supposed to protect women from cognitive decline was found to do the opposite. However, it is essential to note that the results of this trial applied only to women over sixty-five who were taking the estrogen/progestin combination Prempro.

Hormones play a valuable role in the health of the brain. Studies demonstrating the positive effects of hormones on cognition are numerous. When a woman's hormone levels decline at menopause some of the first symptoms she may notice are memory lapses and/or foggy thinking. Estrogen plays a vital role in brain health. Numerous and compelling studies have shown that women who begin hormone replacement at the time of the menopausal transition dramatically reduce their risk of Alzheimer's disease. The women evaluated in the WHIMS trial were all well beyond menopause. This raises an important question: Could a valuable window of opportunity for brain protection have been missed because replacement therapy was not started early enough? In addition, WHIMS only examined the use of one form of HRT, the combination synthetic progestin and animal-derived estrogen product Prempro. What the study did not reveal was what would have happened to these women had they been given a different form of HRT earlier. As with the estrogen-only arm of the WHI trial, the Premarin-only arm of WHIMS is still ongoing. Results will be forthcoming.

The Women's Health Initiative was a massive undertaking. It brought international attention to women's health care and hormone replacement therapy. In spite of the fact that some of the findings were negative, it was a major accomplishment. In science, negative findings can yield positive outcomes. They can tell us that what we have been doing isn't right and force us to do more research, to move in new directions, and to open our minds to better, safer, more effective methodologies. Do the results of the WHI really mean that all women should forgo hormone replacement completely? We think not.

The body has an innate knowledge of how much of a hormone it needs in circulation at any given moment. That's why if there isn't enough of a hormone, as often happens during menopause, when hormone production can begin to decline, women experience symptoms.

The body is struggling to work as effectively as it did when levels were ideal.

The body's hormonal balance is very delicate. It can take only the minutest amount of a hormone to perform its function in the body. If there is too much of a hormone in circulation—an imbalance that can occur if a replacement hormone is given when it is not needed or is given in a dosage that is too high—the body begins to overreact, which can lead to bloating, breast swelling, headaches, and mood swings, or maybe even increased risk for disease.

The hormone levels of the women of the WHI were not tested before the trial began, nor were their hormone levels monitored during the study to determine how they were being affected. Most people don't know that 42 percent of the participants on Prempro actually stopped taking it before the end of the trial. This is not an uncommon occurrence among conventional HRT users. Many women who take standardized doses of synthetic and animal-derived hormones do stop using them after a short time, often because they are experiencing the side effects that come with too much of a hormone, a hormone that is not needed, a hormone that is unfamiliar to the body, or a hormone that belongs to another species. Individualized HRT—knowing what you need, taking it in the most natural form and the lowest dose necessary, and monitoring your response—is the only way anyone should take hormones.

If you are a perimenopausal or menopausal woman who is experiencing symptoms such as hot flashes, night sweats, loss of libido, forgetfulness, depression, anxiety, irritability, or insomnia, and symptoms are affecting your quality of life, you might benefit from hormone replacement. If you are a woman who has had a hysterectomy and your body is no longer producing its own sex hormones, you may need hormone replacement. If you are a woman who has been frightened by all the controversy surrounding HRT, you may not know the whole story. If you are a woman who has any questions at all about hormone replacement, you owe it to yourself to read this book.

Individualized, natural hormone replacement therapy is a choice you need to know about—and it's a choice you have. One of the most important decisions you can make regarding your health is whether to take hormone replacement. Is it right for you? We hope this book will help you to make that decision.

PREFACE

When I graduated from the University of Wisconsin Pharmacy School in 1978, many women who were being treated for symptoms like anxiety, depression, mood swings, bloating, and food cravings were given tranquilizers, antidepressants, and diuretics. They were told that what they were experiencing was "all in their heads." However, many of these women knew intuitively that something was happening with their hormones. Their symptoms seemed to be associated with their monthly menstrual cycles. During certain times of the month they were fine, but over the course of the month their symptoms would escalate, build to a crescendo, and then hit a peak. Once menstruation began, the symptoms would diminish and then disappear.

I listened carefully to these women, to their intuition and wisdom about their own bodies, and I realized they were indeed suffering from something hormonal. I began to question the treatment option of "Here, take this every day and see me in a month," that was being offered to them. If their problems were hormonal, then treatment with Valium was not going to solve them. This was the beginning of my search for a better understanding of the nuances of hormonal fluctuation.

In Europe at that time, premenstrual syndrome, or PMS, was a medical diagnosis, and progesterone therapy was conventionally prescribed for it, in either suppository or injectable form. In America, premenstrual syndrome was not considered a real diagnosis, and progesterone was available only in injectable form. The injections were painful and not very practical for daily use. I began visiting medical and pharmacy school libraries to research and learn as much about progesterone and PMS as I could. Working with women's doctors, I was soon formulating natural progesterone treatments for women who suffered from these hormonal symptoms, and they worked. Women were telling me that they had begun feeling like themselves again.

Gradually, by word of mouth, women heard of the work I was doing and began calling from all over the United States. One woman became 50 women became 500 women, all with questions and concerns about the role their hormones were playing in how they felt. It was a grassroots effort that spread PMS education from woman to woman across the country. I learned a great deal during this time about how women share information, communicate with one another, and learn from one another. And on April 12, 1982, I founded Madison Pharmacy Associates, the first pharmacy specializing in women's health.

We worked closely with women and their doctors, gradually unraveling more and more of the mysteries of women's hormones. It was medicine and pharmacy being practiced the way they were meant to be. It was an exciting and transformational time in women's health care.

By looking at daily symptom records, recording when symptoms occurred and what their intensity was, noting when they were present and when they were not, I found over and over again that every single patient was different. I discovered that some women had specific symptoms that came only at certain times of the month, while other women had symptoms that troubled them every day and then got even worse just before menstruation began. Others recorded having symptoms only after eating certain foods, drinking alcohol, taking a medication, or going too many hours between meals. Still others had symptoms that occurred regularly every other month or every two months, or that became unbearable only at specific times of the year and that varied according to season. There seemed to be more to the story of hormones than we ever imagined.

In the early days of hormone balancing, progesterone was generally prescribed in suppository form. In many cases, within an hour to an hour and a half of using their medication, patients would tell me how much better they felt, often saying they felt like a cloud had lifted. Many women who had been treated with tranquilizers and antidepressants were able to stop taking them and to function normally and quite happily. But that was just the beginning of what I was to discover about hormones.

Over the years, by working with thousands of patients and physicians and studying the effects of natural hormone replacement therapy, I became acutely aware of the individuality of women and the extreme variations in their hormonal needs. In one woman, it might take as much as 400 milligrams of progesterone to create a response, but in another that amount was too much. Some women needed as little as 25 milligrams. Having only my sense of observation to rely on, I started recording all the subtleties of absorption and metabolism I was seeing in my patients. And I began to refine the way in which I formulated hormones. I encouraged physicians and other health-care providers to consider individualizing hormone doses as well. When treatments were individualized, women's responses were infinitely better. I knew I was approaching hormone replacement in a whole new way, but I knew it was the right way. What I needed was a scientific method to verify what I was observing.

And then, because of the work and the research being done at Aeron LifeCycles Clinical Laboratory in California, under the direction of John Kells, I was introduced to saliva testing for hormones. Saliva testing is a scientifically accurate way to confirm what I had been observing about the individuality of a woman's hormonal landscape. My collaboration with John has been like taking a lid off a box and being able to look inside. Through this technology, we can now see exactly how a woman changes hormonally over time, and we can get a true picture of how, as an individual, she responds to hormone replacement therapy. This is an exciting advance in women's health care.

This is what *The HRT Solution* is all about. We want women to know that conventional, one-size-fits-all, synthetic hormone replacement is not their only option. We want women to know that many of the side effects of hormone replacement come not from the hormones as such, but from the random and often excessive way in which they are prescribed. We want women to know that hormone replacement can be both a beneficial experience and an enjoyable one.

—MARLA AHLGRIMM

WHEN ADELINE HACKETT was a little girl in Saskatchewan, Canada, she loved to wander around the large farm she lived on. Her father told her to mark her way home by looking to the horizon, where a large windmill stood. When Adeline grew up and became a scientist, she equated the windmill with the horizon of scientific discovery. In 1986, Dr. Hackett and I founded Aeron LifeCycles Clinical Laboratories. When we named the company, we stretched our scientific imagination to a windmill of the future, an aeron. It symbolized to us the direction we were heading in. It was our intention at that time to speed up the rate of scientific discovery in the area of breast cancer and to bring forth treatments that would help women, both those at risk for breast cancer and those who already had it. Dr. Hackett and Dr. Helene S. Smith, both well known for their research in breast cancer, together had pioneered a way to actually grow breast-cancer cells outside of the body. It was our hope that studying these cells as they responded to various treatments would enable us to better identify which treatments would be most effective for each patient. This task proved too complicated, however, and our efforts were not successful.

Undaunted by this setback, we began to evaluate the whole spectrum of women's health. The scientific research at that time was telling us that soy foods might play a role in protecting women against breast cancer. Epidemiologists had long recognized that Asian women, who consumed large quantities of soy, had a lower incidence of breast cancer than Western women. Many researchers believed that the key to this lower incidence was soy, particularly the phytoestrogen (plant estrogen) in soy called *genistein*. Our expertise with breast-cancer cells compelled us to expand our study, and in 1993 we were awarded a National Institutes of Health (NIH) grant to study the effect of phytohormones (plant-derived hormones) on breast-cancer cells.

Our studies showed that genistein had the ability to act like an estrogen, but this was in petri dishes, outside the body. Once we found this link, we needed a way to look at what was going on inside the human body as well. We needed a better understanding of the way hormones function and the way they interact with one another. We began to focus our attention on the changes in estrogen and progesterone levels that occur in a woman's body, both day to day and over time. We started to look specifically at the interaction between the "free," or active, hormones and the tissues and organs throughout the human body. To accomplish this, we needed a better and more precise way to measure hormonal changes. This led us to the development of saliva testing for measuring the whole array of sex steroid hormones.

Saliva testing gave us a piece of objective information that had not been available before. It was the true scientific piece of the puzzle we needed to tell us what was happening with a person's hormone levels at that moment. With this ability, our focus then broadened from breast cancer alone to other areas of women's health that are affected by hormonal changes, including menopausal symptoms, cardiovascular disease, and osteoporosis.

We began saliva-testing the hormone levels of a wide variety of individual women. Interestingly, this is when we started learning a great deal about hormone supplements. We found that the way women responded to treatment was very, very individualized. Women who were taking the same hormone replacement formulations were responding differently— the ways in which their symptoms were affected were different, and their hormone levels also were affected in an individualized manner. We could clearly see that giving the same dose of the same hormone to different women elicited individualized responses. Some women responded quickly and dramatically when the hormone entered their system; others had a very slow response. Some required high doses, some much lower doses to restore and balance their hormone levels. Through saliva testing we could see that what had previously been described as "normal" patterns were actually quite unique and individual when we looked at each woman separately. We realized that these individual differences could be having a profound impact on the way women were responding to the treatments that were being offered to them. Standard hormone treatments were creating nonstandard responses and were very often inducing the symptoms they were supposed to eliminate.

If a woman continues to have symptoms once she has started hormone replacement therapy, usually a doctor's first response is to prescribe a higher dose of the treatment. Of course, the patient's condition will only continue to worsen if her hormone levels are increased when reducing them is what is called for. Being able to accurately test a woman's hormone levels helps her health-care practitioner determine if what she is feeling is based on levels that are too low or too high. We now have scientific information that verifies why a woman responds to HRT in a particular way.

We believe that a very important aspect of the future of women's health care lies in individualizing hormone treatments. It is our mission to change the way physicians think about hormone replacement, and we want to assist them in prescribing it in a safer, more effective, and more rational way.

Based on our experience with thousands of women, we believe that hormone supplementation should be monitored in order to provide long-term health benefits for women while minimizing their risk of adverse effects, including breast cancer. We want to change the way physicians prescribe hormones so that, first, they measure hormone levels before prescribing therapy and then measure hormone levels after therapy has begun in order to customize the treatment to a woman's needs. This is an entirely new approach to hormone replacement therapy.

Our knowledge about hormones is increasing almost exponentially. We are beginning to gain a very deep appreciation of the many ways hormones affect disease and the role they play in our wellness and longevity. Saliva testing of hormone levels is not new. Individualizing prescription medication isn't new, either. But combining these two things and applying them to hormone replacement therapy is new, and what it gives you is a customized form of therapy that takes your individual needs into account in a way never done before. Individuality is the ultimate dimension in hormone management.

—JOHN M. KELLS

The classic definition of a hormone is a substance which travels from a specific tissue where it is released into the bloodstream to a distant responsive cell where the hormone exerts its characteristic effects. What was once thought of as a simple voyage is now appreciated as an odyssey, which becomes more complex as new facets of the journey are unraveled in research laboratories across the world.

—LEON SPEROFF, M.D.

Individualized Natural Hormone Replacement

When most of us go to the doctor, we believe we are getting individualized care. After all, the only people in the examining room are you and the doctor. The doctor listens to *you*, examines *you*, and evaluates how *you* are doing. He or she then prescribes a course of action. Maybe it's simply a date for a reexam, or a lifestyle modification, or it could be a prescription for medication—your own individual prescription. But is this prescription individualized specifically for you? Generally it is not.

While it might be true that your visit with the doctor is your own, the medical treatment you receive is often the same treatment that everyone else who has your same condition receives. Almost all medical prescriptions are written for standardized doses in standardized forms. For example, if you have a very painful ear infection, you will most likely be given a prescription for 500-milligram antibiotic pills. This dose is given whether you are a short, slender, sixty-three-year-old woman or a tall, muscular, twenty-year-old male basketball player. Many women who are given prescriptions for hormone replacement therapy experience this same phenomenon.

Conventional hormone replacement generally consists of standardized doses of synthetic or animal-derived hormone preparations. Whether women are short or tall, heavy or thin, active or sedentary, or forty, fifty, sixty, or seventy years old, they are all given the same prescription—one-size-fits-all HRT, utilizing synthetic and animal-derived hormones. These drugs, while patented and FDA-approved, are not the same as human hormones. They are similar and can fool the body by acting like human hormones, but they are not the same. What's more, conventional dosages of synthetic hormones are often much higher than necessary, which can result in both short-term and long-term side effects. We think there is a better way—individualized, low-dose, natural hormone replacement therapy. In this chapter we are going to tell you why.

YOUR HORMONAL PROFILE: AS UNIQUE AS YOUR FINGERPRINT

Think for a moment about all of the women you know—how they look, dress, walk, talk, and even think. Isn't it amazing how different they are? A whole variety of hair and eye colors, facial shapes and complexions, heights, weights, shapes, and sizes—even identical twins have subtle differences between them that define their individuality. Every woman is her own unique self. And every woman is a hormonal individual, too.

Roberta, Serena, and Melinda are all forty-nine years old and are no longer experiencing menstrual cycles. They are similar in height and weight, and they all enjoy about the same amount of regular aerobic exercise. However, that is where their similarities end. Roberta is experiencing hot flashes and insomnia, and Serena has mood swings. Melinda has no menopausal symptoms at all. Hormone level tests reveal that each of these three women is producing different amounts of estrogen. Serena's estrogen level is well below the range expected for a menopausal woman, Roberta's is only slightly below the menopausal range, but Melinda is still producing the same amount of estrogen she produced when she was much younger. Even though these women are the same age, they are all hormonally different.

Every woman's hormones are produced according to her own biochemistry. Her hormone levels can fluctuate and change daily, weekly, monthly, and from year to year. Her genes, physiology, lifestyle habits, stress level, diet, and even the extent of her exercise can influence them. This is why each woman's hormonal profile is so unique. It's also the reason that some women have regular, uncomplicated menstrual cycles and others have difficulty with premenstrual syndrome (PMS). It's why some women seem to slip through menopause with barely a flutter while others are plagued with hot flashes, night sweats, insomnia, mood swings, dry skin, food cravings, memory loss, and/or fatigue as they go through "the change." Hormonally, women are as distinctly individual as they are in every other way. So what happens when you give women who are hormonally different the same prescription for HRT? It's simple: They all respond in their own way.

RESPONDING TO HRT

Taking estrogen can literally wipe away the sleeplessness, hot flashes, mood swings, and confusion that often come with menopause. But too much estrogen can cause you to have mood swings or make you feel bloated, anxious, and forgetful—even put you at a higher risk for breast cancer. Replacing progesterone can eliminate irritability, calm anxiety, and put an end to mood swings. But too much progesterone can make you feel fatigued and sleepy. Taking dehydroepiandrosterone (DHEA) can make you feel completely energized and young again. But taking too much DHEA can raise your DHEA level too high and can also elevate your testosterone level. For some women, supplemental testosterone can alleviate such symptoms of menopause as depression, diminished sex drive, and bone loss. But using too much testosterone can cause oily skin, acne, an increase in facial hair, or feelings of anxiety and aggression. If you give a woman a hormone she doesn't need, or too much of one she does need, her response may be the opposite of what you hope to achieve.

Your body is like a galaxy of interrelated systems designed to work cooperatively to keep you functioning optimally and in the best of health. Your diet, exercise, emotions, and stress level can all affect how your hormones are processed. For example, a high-fat diet can make it harder to eliminate estrogen from your system. A high-fiber diet can make it easier. The amount of time a hormone stays in circulation can greatly influence how you feel.

The interplay between you and the hormones you take determines how you respond. Some women absorb replacement hormones quickly; others very slowly. Some women metabolize them efficiently; others recirculate and reuse them. This, too, can be influenced by many factors. For example, your body's chemistry is designed to metabolize hormones (break them down and eliminate them) once their job is complete. This is accomplished by means of enzymes. Synthetic and animal-derived hormones are harder to metabolize than your own hormones because they are unfamiliar to your body's enzymes. These foreign hormone molecules stay in your body longer, sometimes causing it to overrespond, which in turn can result in side effects and physical discomforts. Natural replacement hormones are identical to human hormones. Your body recognizes them and metabolizes them just like they were your own hormones.

Hormone replacement therapy is very complex. Not only are women's responses to replacement hormones highly varied, but replacement hormones themselves are very diverse. Different hormonal delivery systems work differently in the body, too. How you take hormone therapy—whether in pill, cream, gel, patch, or suppository form—can dramatically affect how you respond as well. Patches, creams, and gels, for example, are well absorbed and can dramatically reduce—by as much as ten times—the dosage a woman needs to take to manage her symptoms. Tablets and capsules, on the other hand, take longer to metabolize and lose much of their potency as they pass through the liver. In addition, it makes a difference if you take a hormone preparation once or twice a day, in the morning or at night.

The specific type of replacement hormone you take, how much of it you take, when you take it, and the form in which you take it—all have an impact on how your replacement therapy works for you. When you consider all of these variables, doesn't it just make sense to design a woman's hormone replacement to meet her specific needs?

WHAT'S RIGHT FOR YOU?

Symptoms are good indicators that your hormone levels may be low. But symptoms alone won't tell you *which* of your hormone levels are low or exactly how low they are. Some women experience hot flashes because they have low estrogen, but some experience them because of low progesterone. If a woman takes estrogen when she doesn't need it, she is going to experience side effects. Rather than getting rid of her hot flashes, too much estrogen can actually make them worse.

As many as half of all women who are hormonally out of balance, or who are in perimenopause or menopause, have no outward signs. Even though they are not experiencing symptoms, their hormone levels may still be low enough to put them at risk for "silent" diseases like osteoporosis and other chronic degenerative diseases commonly associated with aging. If you were in this situation, how would you determine whether you were a candidate for hormone therapy? Testing your hormone levels is really the only way to know for sure if your hormone levels are low.

To truly benefit from hormone replacement, you have to know exactly which hormones you need, how much of each you should be taking, and how you are responding to them once you start. The only way to do that is to test and monitor your hormone levels. There are simple hormone-level tests that are easy to take and can be done in the privacy and comfort of your own home. They can tell you and your health-care practitioner exactly what your hormone levels are and which hormone or hormones (if any) you need, which can help to establish how much of each you should be taking.

There are also methods of formulating and customizing hormone prescriptions so they meet your needs in the lowest dose necessary to achieve relief of symptoms. Pharmaceutical companies have recognized that a woman's body responds very well to natural hormones; consequently, there are new natural hormone products coming on the market all the time. However, these products are still offered only in one-size-fits-all standardized doses. The more we work with women to meet their individual needs, the more keenly aware we become of how minute replacement hormone dosages can be and still be effective. A very little goes a long way when it comes to hormones.

Once you begin therapy, monitoring your hormone levels tells you exactly how you are responding. If your symptoms are abating but your hormone levels are above the expected range for a woman your age, then your dosage can be adjusted down. There is never a reason to take more of a hormone than you need. There are also other tests available that can tell you how your therapy is working. Bone-resorption tests such as the urine deoxypyridinoline (Dpd) test measure your rate of bone loss. These are simple urine tests that can also be done in the privacy of your own home. If you begin taking hormone replacement to prevent bone loss, you can monitor how effective it is with a follow-up Dpd bone-resorption test. If your rate of bone loss has slowed, you know your therapy is effective. Tests such as the Dpd have helped confirm that replacement hormones can be effective at very low dosages—as much as one-tenth to one-twentieth of those that have commonly been prescribed. Hormone level assessment combined with bone-resorption testing can tell you whether you need to adjust your hormone therapy. It takes the guesswork out of HRT.

Throughout your life, your hormones increase and decrease, fluctuate, and change. They are with you from the time you are born until the moment you die. We like to think of the journey you take with your hormones as your hormonal river of life. What is happening with you hormonally at any given time can have a great impact on how you feel and how your body functions. Knowing exactly where you are on your hormonal journey can help you to make important decisions about your health and well-being.

THE CHOICE IS YOURS

Women are living longer today than ever before. Did you know that if you live past your fiftieth birthday, you can reasonably expect to live well into your eighties? That means you will spend nearly half of your life in perimenopause, menopause, and postmenopause. What a thought! Living a long life is an enticing prospect, but how often do you hear someone say, "Sure I want to live to be 100, but only if I am healthy"? And it is so true. We all want to go the distance feeling healthy, strong, and sharp. Our quality of life is as important as the quantity. Along with recharging your batteries and slowing the aging process, some of the most important reasons for using hormone replacement are to stop bone loss and to protect you from many of the degenerative diseases that seem to come with age.

We want you to know that natural hormones that are identical to your own are a choice you have. We want you to know that individualized hormone dosages designed specifically to meet your body's needs are a choice that you have. And we want you to know that hormone-level testing to monitor your therapy is a choice you have. Cookie-cutter HRT is not all there is.

For over twenty years, individualized, natural hormone replacement therapy has been improving the quality of life for countless women and protecting many of them from chronic and debilitating diseases. The information in this book about this form of hormone replacement will empower you with the knowledge you need to take charge of your health. Each chapter will give you new insight into why it is such an important choice. So let's get started.

In order to make the most informed decisions about protecting your health, you have to understand how your body works. For centuries hormones have been the brunt of wisecracks and jokes. How many times have you heard someone say that a woman's emotions or sensitivities are simply her hormones acting up? But hormones are no joke. In the next chapter you'll discover how powerful they really are. Just about everything that goes on in your body is in some way influenced by your hormones.

2

HORMONES 101

Soon after her twelfth birthday, a young girl begins a monthly hormonal cycle that will last for nearly forty years. She may be told fairly early on that it is the actions of the hormones estrogen and progesterone that cause her menstrual cycles to begin. When she gets a little older and goes through puberty, she will probably find out that another hormone, testosterone, is responsible for all the differences between "Venus" and "Mars." But, in reality, those are only a few pieces of a woman's hormonal puzzle.

From the very beginning of your life, your hormones govern much of who you are. They are with you from the moment you are conceived. They define whether you are male or female, and, it is now believed, they help to define how you look, how you feel, how you think, how you behave, how you age, and even whether you are healthy. In a complex and intricate dance, your hormones circulate throughout your bloodstream, carrying messages as simple as "go to sleep" and as profound as "begin the miracle of birth." These powerful substances are found virtually everywhere in your body: in the tissues of your brain, your gastrointestinal tract, your reproductive organs, your kidneys, your liver, and—amazingly—even in your saliva.

Hormones circulate throughout your body and control just about everything that goes on. Each hormone has a specific job to do. Yet hormones also work together, affecting and communicating with one another in ways that are remarkable and mysterious.

Just what are these amazing things called hormones? In order to navigate your hormonal river of life successfully, you have to understand just that. In this chapter, we are going to introduce you to the basics—what hormones are, what they do, and how they do it.

WHAT ARE HORMONES?

The classic definition of a hormone is "a chemical substance that is produced in one location in the body and travels to another to create a response." Most hormones begin their lives in endocrine glands. The pituitary, thyroid, parathyroid, pineal, and thymus glands, as well as the pancreas, adrenal glands, and ovaries (or testes) are all endocrine glands. Together, they make up your endocrine system. Your stomach, small intestine, liver, kidneys, and brain can also make hormones, but for now we are going to focus on the endocrine glands, glands whose sole function is to produce hormones. Much as a finely trained surgical team works together, elements and enzymes come together in the endocrine glands and produce hormones.

Your endocrine system is the cornerstone of your health. It manages and controls everything from your immune response to your energy output. For example, it regulates your blood-sugar level, maintains the crucial balance among your body's electrolytes (important minerals like sodium, potassium, calcium, and magnesium), and enables you to build strong, healthy bones. It determines how you mature and how slowly or quickly you age. Thanks to your endocrine system, you are able to become pregnant and carry a baby if you choose. Your endocrine system helps you to digest and assimilate your food, convert it into energy, and then use the energy to build muscles or burn fat. And remarkably, your endocrine system monitors not only what is going on inside you but also what's going on around you. It interprets what you see and experience, and translates it into physical reactions in your body, enabling you to adapt to change and to cope with stresses of all kinds.

How does it do all this? With powerful chemical messengers called *hormones.* Hormones tell your cells what to do. They are the sparks that make things happen. They turn things on and turn things off, turn things up and turn things down. Your thyroid hormones regulate and monitor the rate of your metabolism. If you have too much glucose (sugar) in your blood, the hormone insulin, secreted by the pancreas, helps to decrease it; if you do not have enough, adrenaline from your adrenal glands increases your metabolism of carbohydrates to supply the needed glucose. If you have too much calcium in your blood, the thyroid hormone calcitonin helps to lower it. The sex hormones estrogen and progesterone control the rhythm of your monthly cycles. Estrogen and another sex hormone, testosterone, wake up your libido. Dehydroepiandrosterone (DHEA) helps you to create and maintain lean muscle mass. At night, the pineal hormone melatonin helps you fall asleep. And the list goes on. There is seemingly no end to the work your hormones do.

YOUR BODY'S INFORMATION SUPERHIGHWAY

You can think of your endocrine system and your hormones as your body's great information superhighway. In much the same way as a message is sent from one computer to another, your endocrine system and its hormones are the means by which messages are sent over long distances in your body, from your brain to your glands and organs, from your nervous system to your fingertips and the end of your nose.

Many people think of the nervous system as the body's only internal communications network. In fact, if your body had only its nervous system to rely on as a communications network, you would have to have millions more nerve cells than you do. Nerves communicate messages using a kind of relay system, moving messages along from one nerve to another. For example, if you cut your finger, in order for your finger to send an SOS call for assistance, nerve endings have to be right there, near the cut. And they are—that's why you flinch and say ouch! The nerves in your finger pick up the injury message and send it immediately through your nervous system to your brain.

Once your brain gets the message that you have a wound, it sends an alarm to your endocrine system that places your entire body's defenses on red alert. Right away, the hormone adrenaline gets pumped into your bloodstream to give you the energy you need to cope with your injury and to run for help if you have to. Then another adrenal hormone, cortisol—the stress hormone—comes rushing in to help reduce any inflammation or pain that might arise because of the wound. To protect the wound from infection, DHEA alerts your immune "troops" to the possibility of bacterial or viral invaders. And that's just some of what goes on.

HOW IT WORKS

Let's take a closer look at exactly how this whole hormonal information superhighway actually works. An endocrine gland produces a hormone and sends it into your bloodstream, carrying a specific message. But the message is written in a kind of chemical code. So in order to deliver the message, the hormone has to find a cell that understands its code. These message-receiving cells have *receptors,* and they are found virtually everywhere in your body—in your brain, digestive system, bones, breasts, lungs, eyes, and even your heart. Receptors interpret the messages that hormones are sent to deliver. In order to deliver its message, a hormone must bind with the appropriate receptor. Once the hormone binds with the receptor, it is transported into the nucleus, or message center, of the cell, where the message gets decoded and the job the hormone has been sent to do begins.

Each hormone has specific jobs to do and specific places in your body to do them. Where a hormone goes and what it does depends on which receptor is its target and what that particular receptor is coded to interpret. For example, an estrogen molecule can bind with receptors in your bones and decrease bone loss, or it can bind with receptors in your brain and enhance your memory. Testosterone can bind with receptors in your brain and awaken your libido, or it can bind with receptors in your skin, where it can increase oil production.

Each hormone has its own receptors. And even though an individual hormone may have different jobs to do in different locations in the body, it has to connect with one of its own receptors to create a response. In other words, an estrogen molecule will not turn on a testosterone receptor (or vice versa). The relationship between hormones and their receptors is very specific.

The way in which a hormone fits with its receptor is exact, like a key fitting into a lock. You can think of it this way: You are at the car dealership to buy a new car. You pick out a brand-new white Toyota Camry, fill out the papers, and give the salesman his money. In return, he hands you the key. When you step outside, you are faced with hundreds of Toyotas, many of them Camrys. At least twenty-five of them are *white* Camrys. Yet even though they all look alike, there is one unique thing about one of them, and it's in your hand. That key you're holding will open only the door of your new car and none of the others.

When a hormone binds with its receptor, one of two kinds of responses can result. One is immediate—in other words, it happens right away. The other is a response that occurs over time. For example, if an estrogen molecule leaves your ovary and goes to your brain to clear your mind and sharpen your focus, your response can be swift. On the other hand, if an estrogen molecule tells your breast cells to get ready for a baby that's coming, the response may take a few days or even weeks.

After a hormone has entered a receptor and its mission has been accomplished, the hormone is no longer necessary. A team of enzymes then comes along to metabolize it (break it down). This process of hormone metabolism also is exact and specific. Hormone enzymes recognize the hormones they are designed to work on, and they bypass ones that are not familiar to them. The by-products that result from the metabolism of hormones are called *metabolites*. Some metabolites are useful (even essential); others are waste products that are meant to be eliminated. How efficiently hormones are metabolized can have a great impact on how you feel.

HORMONE PRODUCTION AND REGULATION

When it comes to hormones, your body seems to know just how much of each one it needs in order to function optimally. And when it comes to regulating those amounts, your body relies on some very complex systems of checks and balances.

Some hormone levels follow a regular daily clock, rising and falling at the same time each day. For example, the pineal gland releases melatonin into your system at about the same time every day. Your melatonin level is generally higher at night and lower in the morning. If it weren't, you would probably have trouble falling asleep, because melatonin tells your body when it is time to go to sleep.

Some hormones are released into your system automatically and predictably. They are always produced at the same intervals. The interval can be every few minutes, every few hours, or even every few weeks. Estrogen and progesterone function this way. With synchronicity and regularity, they work together to manage your fertility cycles. This is what enables your reproductive system to be (at least) as reliable as it is.

Some hormones are released when the need arises—for example, if you are injured, fall ill, or become pregnant. Your endocrine system is constantly evaluating what is happening to you and deciding what you need in order to manage it. If you come down with the flu, your hormones are there to help you get well. Or if you develop something more serious than the flu and have to take potent medications to get better, your hormones are there to help you adjust to the illness and to the impact of the medicine on your system. If a loved one dies suddenly and you are left alone, feeling frightened and isolated, your hormones are there to help you cope with the stress. During holidays and other times of celebration—if you eat too much, drink too much, play too much—your hormones balance your blood sugar, monitor your water retention, even boost your energy to keep you going. If you then decide to go on a diet and start exercising, your hormones are there to help you lose weight and build muscles.

CHECKS AND BALANCES

So your body knows what it needs and when. But how does it control and regulate hormone production so that it gets what it needs, in just the right amounts and at the right time? Again, through a complex system of checks and balances.

Supply and Demand

To begin with, the secretion of a hormone is determined by how much of it is already circulating in your blood. In other words, hormones themselves control their own secretion.

This works much as a thermostat on a heater does. If you set the thermostat at 70°F, every time the temperature falls below 70°F, the heater turns on. When the temperature in the room reaches 70°F again, the heater shuts itself off. Similarly, if you don't have enough of a particular hormone in your system, its production increases. As the amount of hormone rises and gets closer to its optimum level, production slows down. If you go beyond that level and have too much hormone in your system, its production stops.

Bound and Free Hormones

Another important way hormones control their own levels is through a binding process that renders them inactive. Not all hormones are actually destined to deliver their messages.

When hormone molecules are released into your bloodstream, most of them (90 to 99 percent) bind to protein molecules there. These are called *bound hormones*. They provide you with a kind of reservoir of circulating hormones, but they are inactive. In other words, they are unable to bind with receptors and create a response. The hormones that are left "free" (1 to 10 percent)—the ones that do not bind with protein—can bind with your receptors and go to work right away. Free and bioavailable hormones are the only hormones that can actually make something happen.

This system of checks and balances helps to control the amount of free hormone available to your receptors. For example, when your body produces estrogen, your liver increases its production of a specific protein called *sex hormone binding globulin* (SHBG). This is to ensure that some of the estrogen will be taken out of circulation and held in reserve so that you won't have too much of it circulating. The binding of hormones to protein serves as a natural way for your body to protect your receptors from overstimulation.

Protein binding also functions in another way. The protein can bind more tightly to some hormones than to others. This helps to maintain a balance in the ratios between the various hormones. For example, if you have 100 molecules of testosterone and 100 molecules of estrogen circulating in your bloodstream, the binding protein will grab 98 of the testosterone molecules and only 90 of the estrogen molecules. Why? Because some hormones bind more tightly to the binding globulin than others. In your body's system of checks and balances, this is yet another way to ensure that you have only as much of the active forms of various hormones as you need circulating in your body. Women need to have much less testosterone than estrogen in circulation.

Synchronicity

Another way in which your hormone levels are regulated is by the dynamic relationship that receptors have with the hormones. Receptors have built-in feedback mechanisms that control your body's sensitivity to hormones. During your menstrual cycle, for example, when estrogen rises and peaks, your production of estrogen receptors also increases, in turn increasing your body's ability to respond to the estrogen. This is called *up-regulation of the receptors.*

Why does this happen? Because there is a lot of estrogen work that needs to be done during the first half of your menstrual cycle. At the same time this is happening, estrogen also begins priming your body to respond to progesterone by causing your body to increase its production of progesterone receptors. Your progesterone level increases during the second half of your cycle. It's almost as if your body says, "Hey, wait a minute! We can't have all this estrogen floating around without some progesterone, too." Then, when your progesterone level goes up, your body begins *down-regulating,* or decreasing, the number of estrogen receptors so that you are not as sensitive to all the estrogen still circulating in your body.

This kind of ensemble monitoring goes on among all of your sex hormones all the time. In a kind of syncopated rhythm, your hormones up-regulate and down-regulate each other to maintain the balance that is your individual hormonal profile.

In the big picture of hormone production, there is yet another hormonal pattern that dramatically affects your life. It is the rise and fall of your sex steroid hormones. These hormones are often referred to simply as *sex hormones,* but since they also belong to a special class of hormones known as *steroids,* it is more accurate to call them *sex steroid hormones.* The sex steroid hormones, which include DHEA, progesterone, estrogen, and testosterone, are the essence of your vitality, immunity, mental acuity, strength, and sexuality. Cortisol, while not technically a sex steroid hormone, also has an intimate relationship with the sex steroid hormones.

Often called *superhormones,* these hormones are in a class by themselves. In fact, the rise and fall of these potent molecules determines much of what happens to you as you age. In the next chapter, we will see how these powerful hormones work together to protect your health and enhance your well-being.

3

THE RISE AND FALL OF YOUR
SEX STEROID HORMONES

From the moment you are conceived, your sex steroid hormones work together to define whether you are male or female, when you become reproductive and when you stop, how you fight infection, and how well you are protected from disease. Of the myriad hormones, chemicals, nutrients, cells, and substances you have in your body, these hormones seem to determine everything, from how sharp your mind is, to how strong your bones are, to how long you stand straight and tall. How much energy you have, how sexy you feel, even whether you are able to sleep peacefully at night are all determined by this ensemble of characters known as your sex steroid hormones. In this chapter, we will see how your sex steroid hormones all play a role in determining not only *how* you age but also *when* you age.

THE RISE . . .

Birth, which among other things is a monumental hormonal event, marks the beginning of the rise of your sex steroid hormones. Actually, even before you were born, estrogen, progesterone, DHEA, testosterone, and cortisol worked together to help you develop from an embryo into a fetus and then into a baby. Then, as you grew and developed, they changed you in miraculous ways. You got taller, stronger, heavier, and then—in the pinnacle of hormonal excitement called *puberty*—you started your menstrual cycles and became reproductive. This event seemed to hurl you forward with incredible force. Your thinking, your interests, your perceptions, and your feelings all changed. Your body changed, too: Your hips widened and your breasts got larger. Your sex steroid hormones were hard at work. Before you knew it, you entered adulthood. In your thirties, you reached a kind of hormonal peak. You hit your stride, feeling strong, fit, and smart. Life just could not be better.

. . . AND THE FALL

As you round the bend and enter your forties, however, you begin to change again. Your usually predictable menstrual cycle gradually becomes more irregular. You start having that warm-all-over feeling that makes you wonder if you just had a hot flash. Your moods may start to fluctuate. Cranky and irritable for no apparent reason? Possibly. Depressed? Fatigued? Sometimes. Losing interest in sex because it has become too uncomfortable? Frustrating, but true. Exercising like crazy but not feeling as toned? Could be. Craving more caffeine, carbohydrates, and sweets? Probably so. What's going on? It's the fall of your sex steroid hormones.

Lana, 51, is the director of marketing for a large shoe-manufacturing company. Recently, she has been thinking about a career change. An avid horticulturist, she is considering making a leap of faith toward something she has always wanted to do—own a small nursery. Why not? After all, in today's world, entering midlife means you are just hitting your stride.

In many ways, Lana feels inspired to make this change. Her children are grown. She has more freedom now to pursue her own interests. But the truth of the matter is, instead of feeling as if she is hitting her stride, Lana has been feeling as if she's having a hard time just getting up to speed. For one thing, she's been having trouble sleeping lately. Some nights it seems to take forever to fall asleep. Other nights she falls asleep easily but cannot stay asleep, and ends up tossing and turning all night long. In either case, she has trouble waking up in the morning and just doesn't have as much energy as she once did. Even when she is able to sleep at night, Lana sometimes wakes up grumpy for no apparent reason. And if she doesn't wake up feeling grumpy, all those little "changes" she sees staring back at her from the bathroom mirror take care of that. Her skin seems more drawn and tired-looking. She does not feel as attractive as she used to. She has been exercising regularly, but nothing seems as firm as it did even a year ago. And this is just the beginning of her day!

At work, Lana knows she is staring out the window and daydreaming too much, but she can't help it. She doesn't know whether it's because she doesn't like her job anymore or because she is having more difficulty focusing her attention. If anyone asks her what she is thinking about, she often says, "Nothing." And it's true. Whatever it was she was thinking about seems to have flown right out of her mind the minute she was asked. She's even forgotten her PIN at the bank a few times recently. "Maybe my mind is going," she thinks. As her day progresses, Lana finds herself being irritated by little things or, worse, crying about them. She never used to cry so easily, but now, blue Monday seems to have turned into "blue more days than not."

Facing the evening is a challenge, too. Lana just doesn't seem to have the same old zip and zing. When her husband is ready to go to bed, all too often Lana finds herself giving him a little peck on the cheek and telling him to go on without her because she has to catch up on some reading. But this isn't about reading that Lana wants to do; it's more about what she doesn't want to do. Lovemaking just isn't what it used to be. It's not her husband's fault. It's just that somehow, somewhere along the way, her libido left town.

As a woman ages and her body begins to change, she may think to herself, "Uh-oh, my estrogen is slipping away." Like many other women, Lana is beginning to wonder the same thing. But is that all that's happening? Is it only her estrogen that is responsible for the changes in how she looks and feels? Maybe so, but then again, maybe not.

The sex steroid hormones—estrogen, progesterone, testosterone, DHEA, and cortisol—all work together like an ensemble cast of characters. As you know, an ensemble is built on the strength of all the players working as a team, not on any one solo performance. Who would Lucy have been without Ricky, Fred, and Ethel? It's the same with your sex steroid hormones. Each hormone has its own role to play in your health and your aging process, and each one works with all the others. Your sex steroid hormones are a delicately assembled team, and your body strives to maintain a balance among them. As we explore these fascinating molecules, you will begin to see how inextricably they are tied to one another. You will come to realize that, like the ripples that form when a leaf falls into a pond, what affects one can affect them all.

SEX STEROID HORMONES: IN A CLASS BY THEMSELVES

Sex steroid hormones belong to the class of hormones known as steroids, but they have some unique distinctions in their molecular structure that set them apart from other hormones. Their molecules have a characteristic ring-shaped structure. As a result, chemically speaking, they all look remarkably alike. There are, however, slight differences between them. These subtle variations translate into remarkably different effects on the body.

The adrenal glands and the ovaries (the testes in men) make sex steroid hormones, but so can the brain, liver, skin, and even the retina of the eye. And each sex steroid hormone can be made in more than one place. For example, the estrogens can be made both in the ovaries and in the adrenal glands; DHEA can be made both in the adrenals and the brain.

All sex steroid hormones are made from cholesterol. Most of us associate cholesterol with too much steak, but cholesterol is actually an essential building block of these vital hormones. This does not mean, however, that if you have a high cholesterol level, or if you eat food with a high cholesterol content, all that cholesterol is going to turn into hormones. It simply means that cholesterol is the raw material your body uses to make them.

From a molecule of cholesterol comes the precursor hormone pregnenolone. A precursor is a substance or cell from which another substance or cell is formed by natural processes. Thus, a precursor hormone is one that can be converted into other hormones. Pregnenolone is the precursor of all of the sex steroid hormones. But in fact, one distinctive property of these hormones is that each can be transformed into one or more of the others. DHEA, for example, can become testosterone and estrogen; progesterone can ultimately become estrogen, testosterone, DHEA, or cortisol. When this transformation takes place, it is called a *cascade effect* (see Figure 3.1).

The Sex Steroid Hormone Cascade (Simplified)

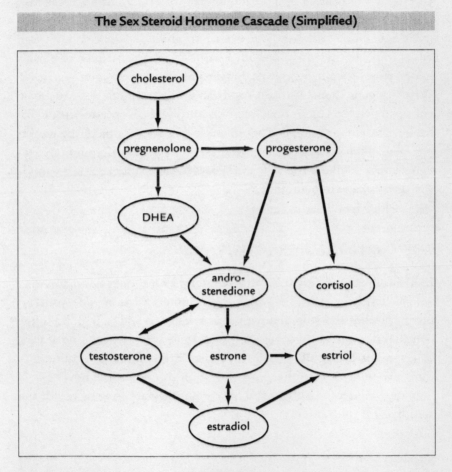

FIGURE 3.1

The origin of sex steroid hormones can be traced back to molecules of cholesterol that are transformed into molecules of the precursor hormone pregnenolone. From pregnenolone, ultimately, come all of the sex steroid hormones. In addition, each of these hormones can be transformed into one or more of the others, as pictured in a simplified form above. This is one of the ways in which your body maintains its hormonal equilibrium.

The cascading of hormones into one another is determined by your body's innate knowledge of what it needs. This is yet another way in which your body maintains its hormonal equilibrium. Fluctuations in your hormone levels can be caused by normal events, from your regular monthly cycle or menopause to stress, illness, and advancing age. When your body needs more of a hormone than is freely available, it can take another hormone and convert it into what it needs. For example, normally your body relies on your ovaries to produce estrogen. However, when you enter menopause—either naturally or because you have had a hysterectomy—your ovaries no longer provide the estrogen you need. What happens then? You still need estrogen. In an effort to maintain your estrogen level, your body can transform DHEA or testosterone that has been stored in your fat cells into estrone. Estrone is one of the weaker estrogens, but it is an estrogen nevertheless. Conversely, if your body recognizes that you have too much of a particular hormone, that hormone can then cascade into another.

THE CAST OF CHARACTERS

Individually and collectively, your sex steroid hormones affect not only your bones, your heart, your brain, your immune system, and your aging process but also your ability to cope with stress and to respond to the demands of your life in some very remarkable ways. By looking at each of these hormones individually and then at the dynamic relationships they have with one another, you will begin to understand how powerfully they influence you and how important they are to your health and well-being.

Estrogen

To begin with, estrogen is not a single hormone, but a category of hormones. Three of the most common forms of estrogen are estradiol, estrone, and estriol. Even though they are all estrogens, each functions a bit differently and at different times in a woman's life. The estrogens are produced predominantly by your ovaries, but they are also produced in your adrenal glands. Though they are generally considered female hormones, they are also produced in small amounts in the adrenal glands in men.

The estrogens are powerhouses of activity. You have estrogen receptors just about everywhere in your body—in fact, they are located throughout your brain, heart, blood vessels, bones, skin, intestines, and respiratory tract, as well as throughout your entire genitourinary system. They affect everything from the way your skin looks and feels to the way your heart beats.

Estradiol is the most active of the estrogens. It is produced mainly by the ovaries. As long as you are having menstrual cycles, it is your estradiol that is doing most of the "estrogen work" that is going on in your body. In fact, throughout the rest of the book, we will be referring to estradiol more often than any of the other estrogens.

Estrone, another of the estrogens, is the one most commonly found in increased amounts in postmenopausal women. The body derives it from the hormones that are stored in your body fat. Estrone does the same work that estradiol does, but it is considered weaker in its effects.

Estriol, the weakest of the estrogens, is produced in large amounts by pregnant women. Women who are not pregnant have small amounts of estriol in their bodies.

For many years, scientists have known that estrogens have a powerful and important influence on health and the aging process, but as research continues, more and more benefits of estrogen are coming to light all the time. For example, researchers have discovered that estrogen is a powerful antioxidant, able to protect the body from damage by free radicals. Free radicals are unstable compounds that can attack and damage healthy cells and tissues. Antioxidants prevent them from doing this.

In matters of the heart, estrogen is a major player in a number of ways. Because of its antioxidant action, estrogen helps to protect the linings of the arteries from free-radical damage, which helps to keep them healthy, flexible, and relaxed so that blood can flow freely through them. Estrogen also increases the body's production of high-density lipoproteins (HDLs, the so-called good cholesterol) that helps to remove low-density lipoproteins (LDLs, or "bad cholesterol") from your system. This means less plaque formation and clogging of the arteries. Estrogen has also been shown to reduce the levels of clot-forming substances in the blood, making it less likely that blockage in a major artery will develop and result in a heart attack.

Exciting research is also revealing the powerful influence that estrogen has on the brain. In the brain, estrogen stimulates the production of choline acetyltransferase. This is an enzyme that stimulates the synthesis of acetylcholine, a brain chemical that makes the transmission of messages from one brain cell to another possible. When acetylcholine production decreases, the storage and retrieval of memories become more difficult. Studies have shown that people with Alzheimer's disease often have only 10 percent (or less) of the level of acetylcholine transferase that is considered normal. Does this mean that estrogen can protect us from Alzheimer's disease? Research suggests that the answer to that question may well be yes.

When it comes to your skin, estrogen supports the production of collagen, the connective tissue that gives structure and tone to your skin. It helps to maintain moisture in your skin by making sure that your body produces enough hyaluronic acid, a substance that helps keep water in your tissues. Estrogen also helps to maintain the strength and elasticity of your vaginal and bladder tissues.

We know that low estrogen levels are associated with a higher rate of bone loss. Even though all of estrogen's actions on the bones are not yet completely understood, we do know that there are estrogen receptors in bone and that the activity of both osteoblasts (cells that build bone) and osteoclasts (cells that break down bone) are affected by estrogen. Estrogen also helps your body to utilize calcium, which in turn helps you to maintain strong bones. This may be the reason that estrogen also helps to protect against cavities and tooth loss. Some researchers believe that, because your teeth are connected to your jawbone by ligaments, it is important for your jawbone to maintain its size and strength in order for you to maintain your teeth. Bone loss and resulting shrinkage of the jawbone can mean a loosening of the tension necessary to hold your teeth in place.

There is seemingly no end to the work the estrogens do in your body. They are stimulating hormones and are very busy indeed. Remember when you were going through puberty, how quickly and dramatically your body changed? Your hips got round, your breasts filled out, and your menstrual cycles started. That is because estrogen was doing what estrogen does—making things happen. But it is possible to have too much of a good thing. Fortunately, nature has provided a perfect plan: Progesterone helps to protect you from the effects of too much estrogen.

Estrogen and progesterone are a dynamic duo in the cast of characters that are your sex steroid hormones. We tend to focus on these potent partners as reproductive hormones, which they are, but their effects are much more far-reaching than that. But before we talk about the important partnership that exists between estrogen and progesterone, let us look a little more closely at progesterone itself.

Progesterone

Progesterone is produced by the ovaries and the adrenal glands in women and, in smaller amounts, in the testes and the adrenal glands in men. One of its most important functions is in the female reproductive cycle. The word *progesterone* means "for gestation [pregnancy]." If it were not for progesterone, pregnancy would be impossible. Progesterone prepares the endometrium (the lining of the uterus) for the implantation of a fertilized egg, then helps to maintain it during pregnancy. It also signals the uterine lining to shed if pregnancy is not achieved. But progesterone is important in other ways, too.

Often called the "feel-good hormone" because of its mood-enhancing and antidepressant effects, progesterone plays an important role in brain function. In fact, there is as much as twenty times more progesterone in your brain cells than in your bloodstream. When progesterone is metabolized, it binds with gamma-aminobutyric acid (GABA) receptors in your brain. GABA is an amino acid that acts as a neurotransmitter (a chemical that conducts impulses between nerve cells) and has a calming effect on your brain. Progesterone and some of its metabolites have been found to be active at GABA receptor sites and thus have a similar effect. This connection between progesterone and GABA at least partly accounts for the fact that optimum levels of progesterone can mean feelings of calm and well-being, while low levels of progesterone can mean increased feelings of anxiety, irritability, and even anger.

Progesterone makes other important contributions to your nervous system in a number of ways. Research shows that progesterone may play a role in the maintenance of the nervous system, the sense of touch, and motor function. It has been found to contribute to the formation of myelin sheaths, which surround, insulate, and protect your nerve cells. In your central nervous system, progesterone plays a role in enabling your nerves to communicate with one another.

Studies indicate that progesterone stimulates the bone-building osteoblasts. This may mean that progesterone is important in helping to maintain the strength of your bones. Animal studies bear this out; progesterone has been shown to enhance the formation of new bone cells.

In addition to its other functions, progesterone can regulate and balance other hormones in a number of ways. In fact, you might say progesterone works a little like a hormonal air-traffic controller. This is something that distinguishes progesterone from many other hormones. Progesterone can recognize when there is too much or too little of another hormone and can cascade into DHEA, estrogen, testosterone, and cortisol. Various cells throughout your body can use progesterone to create other hormones as they are needed. It is therefore easy to understand that a deficiency of progesterone can affect many bodily systems. For example, if you suffer from PMS, low levels of progesterone can mean more symptoms—mood swings, irritability, depression, food cravings, and weight gain. If you are entering menopause, low levels of progesterone can result in intense and very dramatic discomforts, ranging from insomnia and anxiety to night sweats and the loss of your enthusiasm or desire for sex.

Progesterone can also control the action of a hormone by competing with it for its receptor. For example, progesterone can bind with a cortisol receptor and then just sit there. It cannot turn the receptor on, but it can prevent cortisol from turning it on. In this way, progesterone can help block the negative effects of having too much cortisol circulating in your system. Progesterone indeed has many actions. And, as you are about to see, calming progesterone is able to control the excitable estrogens in some very important ways.

The Estrogen-Progesterone Pas de Deux

During your monthly menstrual cycle, estrogen and progesterone work together in a cyclic fashion. During the first half of the cycle, estrogen is on the increase, stimulating the lining of your uterus to grow in preparation for a potential pregnancy. When you ovulate, there is a major pulse of estrogen just before your ovary releases an egg. Estrogen then begins to recede into the background until it drops off to nearly nothing as menstruation begins.

Progesterone, on the other hand, is nearly nonexistent during the first half of the cycle, but during the second half it begins to take over. Following ovulation, a big wave of progesterone is produced, preparing your uterus for the implantation of a fertilized egg. If the egg is fertilized, your progesterone level stays elevated in order to maintain the lining of the uterus during the pregnancy. If not, progesterone drops dramatically, causing the lining to slough off in menstruation. Your progesterone level then goes down. This cycle repeats itself over and over again throughout your reproductive years.

When estrogen and progesterone are in balance, the rhythm of your monthly cycles is regular and relatively pain-free. If, on the other hand, the ratio of these two hormones is out of balance, you can begin to experience various unpleasant symptoms. For example, if you have too much estrogen, it can lead to a greater than normal buildup of the lining of your uterus, and you may experience very heavy menstrual bleeding as a result. If you have too little progesterone, you may have difficulty getting pregnant or you may have dramatic PMS symptoms.

Perimenopause is the period of time when you are approaching menopause. We now know it can start as early as age thirty-five, with subtle hormonal changes, and can last for as long as ten years. During these years, your progesterone levels begin to decline. While this is happening, your body's ratio of estrogen to progesterone is changing. You are producing more estrogen than progesterone, and you may begin to experience some of the consequences of this imbalance. Just as estrogen stimulates breast tissue to grow if you are going through puberty or preparing for a potential pregnancy, it can affect your breast tissue later in life, too. If you don't have enough progesterone to oppose the activity of estrogen, your breasts can swell uncomfortably and even become fibrocystic. Similarly, estrogen stimulates the cells of the uterus to grow as part of your regular monthly cycle. If you are no longer having periods, however, too much estrogen stimulation can lead to endometrial hyperplasia (excessive growth of the uterine lining) and uterine fibroids (benign fibrous-tissue tumors in the uterus).

Look at what else goes on in the estrogen/progesterone pas de deux:

- Estrogen causes an increase in endometrial cell production; progesterone protects the endometrium from this kind of cell growth.
- Estrogen can suppress the action of your thyroid gland; progesterone can enhance it.
- Estrogen increases salt and fluid retention; progesterone works like a diuretic, prompting the body to excrete fluids.

So if there is not enough progesterone to temper the effects of estrogen, you may experience a number of discomforts and may even be at risk for potentially serious diseases.

Progesterone can also temper the effects of testosterone by helping your body decrease excessive testosterone production. Testosterone is an androgen and plays an important role in both men and women. But just as men's bodies produce small amounts of estrogen, women's bodies produce small amounts of testosterone, in their ovaries and in their adrenal glands. Until recently, it was believed that testosterone played a relatively small role in a woman's health. But even though women produce only 10 percent as much testosterone as men do, it is now believed to be vital to their health and well-being.

Testosterone

Sometimes called the "hormone of desire," testosterone has garnered a lot of attention because of its powerful effect on a woman's libido. But that is not all testosterone does. Testosterone is an *anabolic hormone*. Anabolic hormones are a little like carpenters; they help to build strong muscles, bones, and ligaments. When you exercise or experience any kind of stress, your body goes through a tearing-down process. For example, during strenuous exercise, hormones like cortisol break down tissue and extract from it elements that can be used to generate the energy you need for stamina and endurance. In contrast, anabolic hormones like testosterone (and DHEA) help the body to build itself back up.

By the time a woman goes through menopause, her testosterone level has dropped to about half of what it was when she was younger. This can cause a loss of interest in sex as well as fatigue, irritability, depression, aches and pain in the joints, thin and dry skin, osteoporosis, weight loss, and the loss of muscle development. Testosterone replacement during menopause can reignite a woman's libido, restore a youthful level of energy, rejuvenate her, and renew her enthusiasm. New studies are showing that testosterone may play a key role in bone growth and be an important player in the prevention of osteoporosis.

The intimate way in which your sex steroid hormones work together is nowhere more evident than in the relationship between testosterone and estrogen. For example, estrogen primes brain cells to respond to testosterone. In addition, if you do not have enough estrogen in your brain, the testosterone there can cascade into estrogen; if you have too much estrogen, testosterone can desensitize your tissues to its effects. They work together to make sure you can think clearly and have a healthy libido.

Dehydroepiandrosterone (DHEA)

DHEA is the most abundantly produced of the sex steroid hormones. Both men and women produce DHEA, predominantly in the adrenal glands but also in the skin and the brain. And it works with your other sex steroid hormones in many interrelated ways. DHEA can cascade into both testosterone and estrogen, which means that it can come to your aid if those important hormones are fluctuating or in decline. It also has important properties of its own.

A fetus begins manufacturing DHEA during the second trimester of pregnancy. Because DHEA is such a powerful immune stimulant, the expectant mother's body steps up production of it during her pregnancy to further protect the developing child. DHEA also works on the mother's cervix to help during delivery. After birth, it is believed that a baby actually bonds with its mother on the basis of scent, which just happens to be a DHEA-dependent response. DHEA is a precursor to your pheromones, those magical little chemicals that emit your particular scent and act on your brain in response to the scent of others. Could it be that DHEA even influences how you choose your mate?

When you are sick, DHEA aids in your fight against bacterial and viral invasions by mobilizing your immune system to recognize intruders and form antibodies to combat them. It appears to play a role in helping your antibodies remember the invaders so they can identify them during future invasions. This means that DHEA is hard at work protecting you from everything from the common cold to cancer.

Many studies have shown that DHEA helps keep cholesterol in check and plays a role in reducing the formation of fatty deposits in the arteries associated with heart disease. It has also been shown to prevent blood clots and to provide protection against diseases like lupus and diabetes. Research has also determined that DHEA may promote bone growth and reduce a woman's risk of osteoporosis, and it has been shown to be instrumental in weight loss.

Brain tissue contains five to six times as much DHEA as other tissues in the body. DHEA has been shown to improve brain function and cognition, which means that it can help you learn new things, remember them once you have learned them, and answer questions about them when you are asked. Interestingly, people with Alzheimer's disease have been found to have DHEA levels that are approximately half of those found in healthy people of the same age. DHEA can also work as an antidepressant and enhance a person's feeling of well-being. It appears that DHEA plays an important role in maintaining not only a healthy mind but a positive attitude as well.

While most of the research that has been done on DHEA has been in animal studies, more and more human studies are being done all the time. And the evidence is mounting that DHEA is an important hormone that plays a key role not only in how healthy you are and how long you stay that way but also in your overall sense of well-being.

One of DHEA's most important functions is in its role as one of your body's built-in shock absorbers. In much the same way your automobile shocks absorb the hardships of the road, DHEA helps you handle the shocks of life, stresses that could otherwise wreak havoc in your body.

What kinds of stresses are these? Scientifically, as far as the body is concerned, *stress* is defined as a "synergy of endocrinological impairments that creates a syndrome." Loosely translated, that means that stress comes about because you have an effect on your hormones, and your hormones have an effect on you. Sometimes the challenges or circumstances of your life can put a burden on you physically by causing endocrine, or hormonal, events to go on in your body. Medical experts now believe that this is at the root of many degenerative disease processes. In other words, stress has a biological as well as an emotional effect on you, and, over time, it can diminish your body's ability to fortify, protect, regenerate, and heal itself.

Stress can be triggered by emotions, like anger, fear, worry, grief, or guilt. It can be the result of an injury or trauma, an accident, or surgery. An extreme change in diet, exercise, sleep patterns—even the climate you live in can create stress. So can chronic illness, pain, allergies, or inflammation. Too much work, too much play, or too much of *anything* can create stress.

But isn't stress a part of life, and isn't the body supposed to be able to cope with it? Yes. You are born with an innate ability to adapt to the demands of life and even to go beyond your normal limits of endurance when circumstances require you to do so. Your body is designed to re-cover when you are exhausted and to get back up when you are knocked down. But there is more to this equation than you might think.

When you face extraordinary stress of any kind, the hormone corti-sol floods your system. Cortisol is a stress-induced hormone that helps you muster up the energy you need to "fight the tiger." Once you have managed the stressful situation, your brain shuts off the production of cortisol, and DHEA enters the picture to restore calm and bring your body back into balance. In an intimate partnering, DHEA and cortisol work together to help you respond to stress and then to recover from it. But before we go further into how this partnership works, let's take a closer look at cortisol.

Cortisol

Cortisol is produced by your adrenal glands. It is a steroid hormone that belongs to a group called *glucocorticoids.* While cortisol is not technically a sex steroid hormone, we have included it here because of the many important ways in which it interacts with them. Commonly known as the "stress hormone," cortisol helps you to cope with every type of potential stress, from infection to fright, from a heat wave to a divorce. Whether you are at work, at play, or facing an emergency, an accident, or a confrontation, cortisol is there to get you up and get you going.

Cortisol helps determine how the proteins, carbohydrates, and fats from your diet are utilized. For example, cortisol influences the break-down of carbohydrates into glucose so that your body can use them for energy. Cortisol also influences the breakdown of protein into amino acids. Amino acids are the building blocks of protein. They are also the building blocks for your immune system, blood vessels, muscles, and other tissues. Thus, your immune system, blood vessels, and muscles all rely on cortisol for strength and proper functioning. Cortisol prevents the loss of too much sodium from your body and helps to maintain your blood pressure as well. It also helps to suppress bodily reactions such as pain, allergic reactions, and inflammation.

Cortisol helps your body to protect itself from itself. What does that mean? During a strenuous workout, your body breaks down fat and muscle tissue to produce energy. To prevent your immune system from recognizing all of these tissue molecules as foreign invaders, your body produces more cortisol and gently suppresses your immune response so that your body does not go on red alert when it doesn't have to.

The cortisol that can flood your system to assist you in emergencies helps to provide your body with the nutrients you need to cope with stress. That's why it is called the stress hormone. Normally, once you have managed the stressful circumstance, your brain shuts off the production of cortisol, your physical reactions subside, and soon you are back to normal.

Sounds impressive, doesn't it? Well, that's the good news about cortisol. But there is another side of the cortisol story. The bad news about cortisol is that your brain can override messages to shut off cortisol production if it perceives that your stress is ongoing or chronic. Cortisol production then stays elevated because your brain thinks your body needs it to cope with what you are experiencing. And as important and necessary as cortisol is, you can have too much of it. If you have too much cortisol in your system for too long, a damaging cycle can begin that can lead to blood-sugar problems, fat accumulation, compromised immune function, exhaustion, bone loss, and even heart disease.

But didn't we just say that stress is a part of life and that we are meant to be able to cope with it? And that cortisol helps us do that? Yes. But if your stress does not let up—if you are knocked down over and over again—your body grows weary, and before you know it, stress begins to have a detrimental effect on your health. Just like everything in nature, your body is in a continual state of regeneration. It is constantly building itself up, tearing itself down, and rebuilding itself all over again. Your cortisol level goes up to provide you with the energy you need for action. It breaks down tissues in order to do this. Once the job is done, you have to rebuild and recuperate. That is when DHEA comes into play to help you recover so that everything can get back to normal. DHEA and cortisol work together. Under normal conditions, this is the way your body handles your stress.

Cortisol, DHEA, and the Effects of Stress

We all know what an adrenaline rush feels like. We get one when we react to something that excites us, frightens us, surprises us, or makes us angry. An adrenaline rush is the first reaction in a chain reaction of hormonal events. It is the signal that sets in motion the release of cortisol and DHEA into your system. These are the hormones you need to help you take action, to get a job done, even to get your point across. If you are always "under the gun," however—which can mean anything from a continual struggle to make ends meet financially to traveling all the time because you are at the peak of success in your career—then you constantly have stress hormones flooding into your bloodstream. If this happens, your adrenal glands can become overworked and exhausted. Over time, this excess wear and tear on them can be very serious.

The hallmark of adrenal compromise is a decrease in DHEA production. When the buffering effects of DHEA are in short supply or no longer available, then the negative effects of cortisol can go unchallenged. This can leave you more susceptible to everything from hay fever to cancer. Low levels of DHEA are associated with many of the chronic degenerative diseases commonly attributed to aging.

Think about it like this: A fire breaks out in a building. At the firehouse, the alarm bell goes off. The firefighters board their truck and head out to the fire. When they get there, they turn their hoses on and apply all of their energies toward putting it out. When they are finished, they gather up their hoses, clean up the scene, and go back to the station. But what would happen if they didn't turn off their hoses when the fire was out? Eventually, they would flood the scene and one disaster would turn into another. This is similar to what can happen with excess cortisol.

We have learned from studying women who are depressed or experiencing extended periods of psychological trauma that continually elevated levels of cortisol can prevent them from ovulating. If you aren't ovulating, you may not be producing enough estrogen. Low estrogen levels can increase the activity of the bone-metabolizing osteoclasts. To further complicate the situation, in order to provide the extra calcium needed in a fight-or-flight situation, cortisol also stimulates the bone-metabolizing osteoclasts. Left unchecked over a long period of time, high cortisol levels can cause you to lose bone faster than your body is able to rebuild it.

In a natural rhythm, your body produces much more cortisol in the morning than in the evening. This helps you to get up and get started, and also helps you to get through your day. When day is done, your cortisol level should be going down. One study demonstrated that when men come home from work their cortisol levels do go down. This is what is supposed to happen—you come home and wind down. However, the same study showed that many women who work outside the home and have primary responsibility for taking care of their families have cortisol levels that stay elevated in the evening. This is the way their bodies respond to the stress of the "second shift." Women who have high cortisol and low DHEA levels can experience panic attacks and a strange feeling of being both anxious and exhausted at the same time.

Depleted adrenal glands can be at the root of many serious chronic illnesses. As we will see in later chapters, your DHEA and cortisol levels are a very important part of your hormonal profile. Knowing what they are can give you valuable information about how the stresses of your life are affecting your body.

These are your sex steroid hormones. The powerful influences they have on you as you age might make you wonder why, just when you need them, they are beginning to disappear. You would think that because they have such a great impact on us, we would naturally always have them, that our bodies would go on producing them indefinitely. But maybe there is something to that old adage "Youth is wasted on the young," especially when it comes to hormones. It is true that as we age, our sex steroid hormones decline. Do we completely understand why? Not yet. But because we do know they are vitally important to maintaining our health and our sense of well-being, an enormous amount of research is being done on them.

Not surprisingly, your sex steroid hormones seem to be inextricably tied to your reproductive capacity. When it stops, they decline. There is an interesting little wrinkle in this design, however: Although your hormone levels go down, your hormone receptors do not. So if you take replacement hormones, your hormone receptors seem to perk right up and respond. You begin to feel and look younger and have more protection against disease. This is the basis for the practice of hormone replacement therapy (HRT). In the next chapter, we will look at what hormone replacement therapy can do for you.

TABLE 3.1 YOUR SEX STEROID HORMONES AND THEIR BIOLOGICAL EFFECTS IN THE BODY

Hormone	Effects
Estrogen	Protects against osteoporosis, heart disease, Alzheimer's disease, colon cancer, incontinence, and tooth loss and decay.
	Increases the level of serotonin and endorphins as well as other neurotransmitters.
	Enhances sleep, emotional well-being, mental acuity and focus, memory, attention span, communication ability, sensory function (vision, hearing, taste, touch, and smell), digestion, libido, and skin tone.
	Relieves menopausal symptoms and depression.
	Increases tolerance to pain.
	Necessary for fertility.
Progesterone	Has a calming effect.
	Enhances mood.
	Regulates fluid balance.
	Increases energy and libido.
	Balances blood sugar, thyroid function, and mineral balance.
	Necessary for fertility and maintaining pregnancy.
	Relieves menopausal symptoms.
	Decreases risk of endometrial cancer and may help to protect against breast cancer, fibrocystic breasts, and osteoporosis.
Testosterone	Builds muscles and promotes muscle tone.
	Increases energy and libido.
	Enhances sense of well-being.
	Helps to strengthen bone.
DHEA	Helps to protect against heart disease, osteoporosis, diabetes, cancer, Alzheimer's disease, lupus, and rheumatoid arthritis.
	Can increase and enhance energy level, libido, memory, and immunity.
	Protects against the effects of stress.
	Aids in weight loss and healing of burns.
	Helps to prevent wrinkles and dry eyes.
Cortisol	Helps in responding to and coping with stress, trauma, infection, and environmental extremes.
	Increases energy and metabolism.
	Helps to regulate blood pressure.
	Enhances the integrity of blood vessels.
	Reduces allergic and inflammatory responses.

4

THE PROMISE OF HRT

We now know how a woman's body ages hormonally. We know that her sex steroid hormone levels change dramatically from the time she is in her twenties until she is in her seventies and eighties. While a woman is menstruating, she is generally at her healthiest. Her body is producing generous amounts of sex steroid hormones and providing her with important protection against the most serious diseases.

As a woman gets older, her capacity to produce hormones diminishes and her hormone levels begin to decline. This can begin when she is anywhere between the ages of thirty-five and fifty. Whenever it happens, her health risks begin to go up, and it becomes more and more difficult for her body to maintain its hormonal equilibrium. Without enough hormones to go around, she begins to experience symptoms. She may find that she can't sleep, that she wakes up drenched in sweat, that her memory begins to fail her, that she feels depressed, fatigued, and frustrated. She may also find herself getting sick more frequently because her immune system is faltering and steadily growing weaker. Low hormone levels mean that her body may not be getting all the messages it needs to run efficiently. Even if she does not experience symptoms, by the time she is postmenopausal, a woman's risk of developing chronic degenerative diseases like osteoporosis, heart disease, and even Alzheimer's disease has gone up significantly.

We cannot stop the decline of our hormones. Does this mean we are doomed to accept the ravages of time? Not at all, because—perhaps surprisingly—despite the rise and fall of your sex steroid hormones, your hormone receptors do not diminish in their ability to respond to hormonal messages. So just because your estrogen and testosterone levels go down, that doesn't mean your estrogen and testosterone receptors are no longer able to interpret estrogen and testosterone messages. In fact, if a hormone-deficient woman has her hormone levels restored by means of hormone replacement therapy, her receptors seem to perk right up and respond to the messages they receive. Life then goes on just like it always did. Restoring declining hormones can alleviate symptoms of hormone deficiency, reverse hormone-related deterioration processes, and prevent disease.

WHAT'S POSSIBLE WITH HRT

It has been proven that hormone replacement therapy can have a significant protective effect on you and your health as you age. Most specifically, there is undeniable evidence that HRT can have a beneficial impact on your bones and your brain. The scientific evidence regarding heart disease is more controversial, but the final verdict is not in yet. It is important to remember that the two most influential studies that found an an association between increased risk of heart disease and HRT did not investigate the safety or effectiveness of all hormone replacement.

The first and second phases of the Heart and Estrogen/Progestin Replacement Study (HERS and HERS II) and the Women's Health Initiative (WHI) were all designed to evaluate the impact of combination estrogen and progestin therapy (Prempro) on heart disease and quality of life in women. There were 2,763 postmenopausal women participating in HERS and HERS II and 16,000 in the WHI. The findings of both clinical trials pertained to the safety and effectiveness of Prempro.

Interestingly, the average age of the participants in both studies was between sixty-three and sixty-seven. In the HERS II trial, all of the participants had symptoms of cardiovascular artery disease when they en-

tered the study. In the WHI, 8 percent of the women already had a diagnosis of heart disease. In order to determine the true heart- (and
health-) protective power of hormone replacement, it would make more
sense to study healthy women in the age group between forty-five and
fifty-five, before natural hormone levels have declined and disease processes
have begun. The alarming issue underlying the findings of both of these
studies was that the combination of synthetic and animal-derived hormones that had been approved for heart protection was found to have
the opposite effect. The findings simply did not apply to all forms of hormone replacement.

When women go through menopause or undergo hysterectomy and
their hormone levels decline, their risk for disease goes up. Optimum
hormone levels naturally keep us healthier; lower levels put us at risk. Let
us look in detail at three important health concerns and how hormones
affect them.

The Hipbone's Connected to Your Hormones

How often do you think about the importance of your bones? For most
of us, the answer is not very often, not unless something happens to one
of them. But consider this for a moment: Your bones hold your body up.
They support all your muscles, ligaments, and tendons. They are the
framework that gives your body your stature, and, obviously, they contribute greatly to your strength and mobility. Protecting your bones as
you age is therefore a vital aspect of maintaining an active and indepen-
dent lifestyle.

Osteoporosis is a disease in which bone tissue deteriorates because of
a depletion of minerals from the bones. It makes the bones fragile and
susceptible to fracture, and it can strike at any age. If you have osteoporosis, the integrity of your skeleton is compromised because the structure of your bones is breaking down. The weaker your bones become,
the more likely you are to fracture one of them. A person who fractures
one bone is much more likely to fracture another. Osteoporosis is a major health threat for 44 million Americans, over two-thirds of them
women. One out of every two women over the age of fifty will experience an osteoporosis-related fracture at some point in her lifetime.

Osteoporosis is known as a silent disease because it progresses over a
period of years without symptoms. It is often said that by the time you

can feel osteoporosis, you have already fractured one of your bones. The most common cause of bone fracture among older women is a fall. These falls often result in fractured hips, but there can be other fractures as well. For example, if you fall forward and then try to break your fall with outstretched hands, you can fracture a forearm. But osteoporotic fractures are not always caused by something as traumatic as a fall. They can also occur as a result of something as simple as lifting or straining. The most common osteoporotic fractures are those of the hip, spine, and forearm. Hip fractures have the most serious consequences.

Osteoporosis and the fractures that can come with it often cause women to need assistance with the tasks of daily living and even force them into nursing homes, robbing them of their independence and self-esteem. Postmenopausal women have the highest incidence of osteoporosis and the highest rate of deaths attributed to it.

Other facts about osteoporosis include the following:

- There are more than 1.5 million osteoporotic bone fractures a year in the United States alone.
- There are 700,000 osteoporotic vertebrae fractures annually. This type of fracture can bring with it a loss of height, discomfort, and even the dreaded dowager's hump.
- Americans experience a total of 300,000 hip fractures and 250,000 wrist fractures annually, as well as more than 300,000 fractures of other bones.
- Fifty percent of women who suffer fractures as a result of osteoporosis never fully recover.
- One out of every three women who suffers an osteoporotic hip fracture dies within one year.
- By the time a woman is seventy-five, her risk of developing osteoporosis is three times greater than her risk of developing breast cancer.
- Risk factors for osteoporosis include the following: being a Caucasian or Asian woman; a small (thin or petite) body build; an immediate (parent or grandparent) family history of fracture; being estrogen deficient (having gone through menopause, whether naturally or as a result of surgery); being deficient in other hormones, including testosterone, DHEA, and progesterone; a history of taking steroids or thyroid hormones; a sedentary lifestyle; smoking; heavy alcohol consumption (alcohol is toxic to the cells that build bone); a low calcium intake; and

advancing age. Other, less well-known risk factors for fracture include hyperthyroidism; a history of taking medication for arthritis, asthma, lupus, thyroid disorders, and/or epilepsy; the use of antacids that contain aluminum; and excessive caffeine consumption.

We know that estrogen replacement reduces a woman's risk of osteoporosis and bone fracture significantly. Estrogen helps you utilize calcium, the mineral most associated with bone growth. You have estrogen receptors in your bone. Estrogen affects the bone-remodeling process by inhibiting the action of the osteoclasts, the cells that break down bone, and thus helps preserve the strength of your bones. While not all women are at risk for osteoporosis, those who are can significantly protect their bones with estrogen replacement. It has also been shown that women who already suffer from osteoporosis can benefit from estrogen replacement because it can slow down bone loss and help them to preserve existing bone mass.

Exciting new studies are now showing that estrogen replacement may not be the only solution to bone loss. These studies and a great deal of clinical evidence are demonstrating that DHEA, testosterone, and progesterone replacement may all play a role in the health of the bones. The important evidence that hormone replacement can protect your bones should not be ignored.

Every Beat of Your Heart

The health of your bones is not the only reason to consider hormone replacement therapy. Your heart is another. Let us pause for a moment and consider the importance of your heart. This small (about the size of a fist), rhythmically beating organ located near the center of your chest is actually a muscle. And it is the hardest working muscle in your body. Day in and day out, from the time you are in your mother's womb until you die, your heart pumps blood throughout your body. Your heart is the force behind your entire cardiovascular system. Blood pumped by the heart delivers oxygen and nutrients to all the cells and tissues of your body. On its return trip, the blood carries away carbon dioxide and waste materials. If there is a breakdown in this system, the result can be high blood pressure, heart attack, heart failure, stroke, or even sudden death.

Heart disease used to be considered a man's disease, but that is no longer the case. In fact, the statistics on heart disease and women are staggering. Heart disease is the leading cause of death in women over the age of sixty-five. Current statistics show that over the course of a lifetime, women are twice as likely as men to suffer from heart attacks; they are more at risk for a second heart attack; and it takes the average woman longer than the average man to recover from a heart attack. All in all, an estimated 80 million women in the United States are considered to be at risk for heart disease.

Worse, the symptoms of heart disease are subtler in women than in men, so women are often unaware they are at risk until a heart attack strikes. By the time a woman is between the ages of forty-five and fifty-four, her statistical risk of developing heart disease is more than twice as high as her risk for breast cancer. By the time she reaches seventy-five, her risk of heart disease is four times greater than her risk of breast cancer. One out of two women aged eighty-five or older has heart disease. Some of the risk factors for heart disease that you should know about are smoking, family history, a high total cholesterol level, a low HDL ("good cholesterol") level, high blood pressure, increasing age, diabetes, and low estrogen levels.

Science has known for a long time that when estrogen levels go down, heart-disease risk goes up. In fact, as we saw in Chapter 3, many aspects of your cardiovascular system rely on estrogen to keep them healthy and functioning properly. The 1995 Postmenopausal Estrogen/Progestin Interventions (PEPI) study, a clinical trial that included nearly 900 women over a span of three years, demonstrated that women on HRT had better lipoprotein ratios—specifically, higher levels of HDL and lower levels of LDL ("bad cholesterol," which is associated with plaque formation and clogged arteries). They also had lower fibrinogen levels than women not on HRT. Fibrinogen is a component of blood that is involved in the process of clot formation and that, together with LDL, forms plaque in the arteries. High levels of fibrinogen are associated with an increased risk that blockage in an artery will cause a heart attack. The findings of the PEPI trial are significant in furthering our ability to develop and provide better treatment options for women at risk for heart disease.

There are other ongoing studies investigating the role of estrogen replacement in reducing higher than normal levels of insulin and glucose in menopausal women. Both of these are contributing factors to heart disease. The HERS II trial found that taking HRT after menopause prevents increases in fasting glucose levels among women with known heart disease. During the study, 35 percent fewer HRT users developed type II diabetes than did women who were not taking hormone replacement. All of the study participants who already had a confirmed diabetes diagnosis and were given the HRT showed significant improvement in fasting glucose levels over similar women who were given the placebo.

There are also studies under way to look more closely at estrogen's role as a potential calcium channel blocker, vasodilator, and antioxidant. Calcium channel blockers and vasodilators are substances that help to dilate coronary arteries. If you have atherosclerosis (hardening of the arteries due to fatty plaques), the ability of your coronary arteries to expand, and to remain open enough for blood to flow through them and reach the heart, is very important. If an artery is clogged or injured, when it contracts it can become small enough to cut off blood flow to the heart, precipitating a heart attack.

Estrogen's role in reducing homocysteine levels is also being examined. Homocysteine is an amino acid normally found in the body, but elevated levels of it have been associated with atherosclerosis and free-radical damage to the heart. High levels of homocysteine in turn are associated with certain vitamin deficiencies, especially deficiencies of folic acid and vitamins B_6 and B_{12}.

There is a wealth of positive information available about the effects of estrogen replacement on heart disease. And it is well documented in the scientific literature that when a woman's estrogen levels fall, her risk of heart disease goes up. Without the protection of more youthful levels of estrogen, she is more likely to develop cardiovascular disease. Interestingly, a number of scientific papers analyzing the results of the HERS trials and the WHI study suggest that the findings of increased cardiovascular risk may have been the result of factors other than the estrogen replacement. First of all, many of the participants in both of these studies already had heart disease. Second, the women involved in these trials were all well beyond menopause. They had already lived many years without the protective benefits of estrogen.

Heart disease protection can be viewed in two ways: as the prevention of cardiovascular events, such as heart attacks, or as the prevention of the disease process that can lead to cardiovascular events. Many of the beneficial effects of estrogen act to prevent the disease process. Once heart disease is established, estrogen may no longer be able to exert its protective effect. Thus, it may be possible that estrogen replacement yields the most benefit when it is utilized *before* the disease process starts. We need more studies in this area before we can determine whether estrogen replacement should be ruled out as heart protective.

Furthermore, studies are revealing that estrogen may not be alone in its protective effect on the heart. Again, the delicate interactions of all of your sex steroid hormones may come into play. While it is still too early to say for sure, scientific studies suggest that DHEA, testosterone, and progesterone replacement may also help to maintain the cardiovascular system and ensure that the heart stays strong and healthy.

Command Central: Your Brain

When discussing the benefits of hormone replacement therapy, we cannot forget about the brain. Weighing in at only three pounds, your brain, with its billions and billions of nerve cells, packs a powerful punch when it comes to everything that goes on in your body. In its capacity to send and receive messages, consider and make decisions, and process and synthesize information, the human brain rivals—and in many ways far exceeds—the capabilities of the world's most sophisticated computer. Incredibly powerful and complex, it controls virtually all the activities that go on in your body and that are necessary for your survival. Command Central is in charge of everything from your movement, sleep, hunger, thirst, and sexual activity, to the rhythm of your heartbeat, the familiar contraction and expansion of your breathing, and the ebb and flow of your thoughts.

Your brain also controls your emotions—love, hate, fear, anger, joy, sadness, and many others. What you see, what you hear, what you feel, what you smell, even what you say, are all controlled by some part of your brain. Responsible for running all aspects of your life, your brain is at work every minute of the day and all through the night to make sure that the machinery that is you is in working order. It handles, receives, processes, and remembers millions of messages a day. A monkey wrench in the works here can mean spending your days in a mindless fog of confusion; being unable to remember the names and faces of the people you love; losing control over anger, fear, frustration, and important bodily functions; and sinking into depression and isolation. Protecting the health of your brain increases your chances of growing old with wisdom and grace.

There are scientific data now showing that estrogen replacement can cut the incidence of Alzheimer's disease in half. There are 4 million people with Alzheimer's disease in the United States, and twice as many women as men have it. According to the Mayo Clinic, this number is expected to triple over the next twenty years. One in ten Americans over age sixty-five, and nearly half of those over age eighty-five, has Alzheimer's disease.

Estrogen is needed for proper nerve growth in your brain and for making sure the connections are working correctly. The nerve fibers that transfer information between the right and left sides of the brain need estrogen in order to function properly. When estrogen levels go down, those pathways can begin to suffer. Memory begins to falter, wits begin to dull, focus and concentration begin to blur. That is at least part of what happens in Alzheimer's disease.

Studies suggest that DHEA levels also may be a factor in Alzheimer's disease. Remember, your brain makes DHEA. In fact, you have a higher concentration of DHEA than any other sex steroid hormone in your brain. In addition, women have higher DHEA concentrations in their brains than men do. In the brain, DHEA seems to work as an antidepressant and also appears to play a role in your awareness, perception, reason, and judgment.

As you remember from Chapter 3, your brain can use testosterone to make estrogen when it needs it, and progesterone affects your neurotransmitters. Even though we are just beginning to understand the impact that hormone replacement has on the brain, initial studies and clinical evidence both suggest that sex steroid hormones play an important role in brain health. In fact, as research mounts in this area, it appears we will learn that relationships exist between all of the sex steroid hormones and the brain.

THE GOOD NEWS OUTWEIGHS THE BAD, BUT . . .

There is compelling scientific evidence that hormone replacement may have the power to restore, renew, regenerate, and revitalize virtually every aspect of your life, from immunity and mental acuity to strength and sexuality. Scientific studies have shown that women who use estrogen replacement live longer than women who don't. DHEA supplementation can restore energy and improve immunity. Restoring a woman's progesterone level can renew her sense of well-being, help relieve insomnia, and free her of symptoms of PMS, perimenopause, or menopause. It can protect her from endometrial cancer, and may even help protect her from breast cancer. Women who use testosterone replacement can have their lost libido revitalized and experience relief from depression. Many show an improvement in the health of their bones as well. For menopausal women, there is nothing as effective as hormone replacement for wiping away the hot flashes, mood swings, forgetfulness, and confusion, as well as the dryness that affects their hair, skin, nails, vaginal tissues, and mucous membranes.

After reading all the information in this chapter on the benefits of hormones and hormone replacement therapy, you may be wondering if HRT can actually change the way you age, improve the quality of your life, and increase your lifespan. We believe it can.

Yet, in spite of overwhelming evidence that replacement hormones have a significantly beneficial impact on health, only 15 percent of the women who could benefit from hormone replacement actually use it. As many as 30 percent of the women who are given prescriptions for HRT never fill them. About 20 percent of women who do begin conventional HRT stop within nine months. And the most disconcerting statistic of all: 39 percent of women who have a confirmed diagnosis of osteoporosis stop using HRT after only a short time. If the benefits of hormone replacement are so great, why aren't more people using it? In the next chapter we are going to address that question.

5

WHAT ABOUT THE RISKS?

Hormone replacement therapy dates back more than fifty years. Yet only relatively recently have experts begun to realize that what has been done for many years with conventional HRT has in fact opened the door to a whole new branch of medicine—anti-aging and longevity medicine. Research on hormones is being conducted in laboratories around the world. Many of the findings are positive and suggest that hormones indeed are the keys to our health and well-being. But there is also research that suggests there are risks associated with HRT.

It's true, the Heart and Estrogen/Progestin Replacement Study II trial and the Women's Health Initiative both found an increased risk of heart attack, stroke, blood clots, and breast cancer associated with the use of conventional HRT. All participants in both studies were given Prempro— 0.625 milligrams of conjugated equine (horse) estrogens plus 2.5 milligrams of medroxyprogesterone acetate (synthetic progestin) in a single tablet—or a placebo. This raises some questions. First, did all the participants need these particular hormones, in these doses? And second, do the results mean that all hormone replacement is unsafe, or that all forms of HRT have the same risks found in these studies? In this chapter we are going to answer those questions. But to do that we have to first take a look back at how conventional HRT came to be.

WE'VE COME A LONG WAY: A BRIEF HISTORY OF HRT

The hormone estrogen was first identified in the urine of menstruating women in 1926. In 1928, Ayerst, the predecessor to today's pharmaceutical giant Wyeth-Ayerst, synthesized the first estrogen in the laboratory. Progesterone was identified around the same time, but it wasn't until 1939 that Russell Marker, a well-respected American scientist and chemist, developed a method for synthesizing progesterone from plant substances found in wild yams. The process resulted in a molecule that was identical to human progesterone. Shortly thereafter, Marker discovered that identical-to-human estrogen and testosterone could also be derived from this process. The process was inexpensive and could be used to create unlimited amounts of these natural, identical-to-human hormones. They were called *natural hormones* because they were the same as the ones the body made naturally.

Hormones that are the same as the ones the body produces cannot be patented. In commerce, a patent affords a company the exclusive right to market a specific product. Patents therefore also mean profitability, particularly when people are convinced they need the patented product. Once a company holds a patent on a product, it is more difficult for other companies to sell similar products. They first have to come up with patented products of their own. As interest in hormone therapy grew, pharmaceutical companies realized that, with slight modifications, natural, identical-to-human hormones could be altered just enough to be patented. The results were molecules that mimicked hormone activity in the body to some degree, but not exactly.

In 1942, Premarin, a combination of conjugated estrogens made from the urine of pregnant mares and as many as 200 other chemical constituents, was patented by Wyeth-Ayerst. By the late 1940s, it was being distributed to gynecologists across the country. Industry-sponsored studies started springing up everywhere in an attempt to capitalize on the burgeoning market. In 1952, estrogen was found to improve verbal memory skills in elderly women. As early as 1959, it was shown to protect against bone loss. It seemed like there was no end to the benefits estrogen replacement could confer.

And then came a defining moment in women's health care. In 1966, Dr. Robert A. Wilson, a New York gynecologist, published a book called *Feminine Forever* (M. Evans and Company), in which he described estrogen as the "cure" for menopause. In one fell swoop he identified menopause as a deficiency disease that had previously been overlooked because it had been hidden in the shadows of aging. Estrogen, Wilson claimed, was a virtual fountain of youth for women. It would keep them sexy forever and protect them from the calamity of aging. Almost overnight, millions of women became estrogen users. By 1970, 14 million women were taking standardized, one-size-fits-all doses of Premarin. It was the leader among estrogen replacement products. By the mid-1970s, nearly 30 million estrogen prescriptions were being written each year. By 1975, it was in fifth place among the most frequently prescribed drugs in the United States. (By 1990, it would become number one.) Every woman who was taking it was getting the same "cookie-cutter" prescription—whether her body needed it or not.

Meanwhile, the women's movement was fueling interest in progesterone for its potential as a method of birth control. Large doses of synthetic progestins—synthetic versions of progesterone—were proving to be effective in preventing pregnancy. Then, in 1960, based on the clinical trials of a Catholic gynecologist, Dr. John Rock, another defining moment in women's health care occurred. The U.S. Food and Drug Administration (FDA) approved Enovid, a combination of estrogen and progestin, for use as a contraceptive, and "the Pill" was born. In his book *The Time Has Come: A Catholic Doctor's Proposals to End the Battle over Birth Control* (Alfred A. Knopf, 1963), Rock claimed that Enovid was actually a natural extension of the rhythm method of birth control. In a simple twist of fate, or linguistics, progestins were by association considered natural, a misconception that lingers even today. Many doctors still believe progestins and progesterone are one and the same. They are not.

Progestins such as medroxyprogesterone acetate, the progestin found in Prempro and Provera, are not recognized in the body as progesterone. Progestins are harder to metabolize because they are unfamiliar to your body's enzymes. The molecules stay on your hormone receptors longer, which can result in side effects. Many women who take progestins suffer from bloating, breast swelling, headaches, and irritability.

Nevertheless, during the early 1970s, hormone replacement continued to grow in popularity. An enormous amount of research was being done to investigate the impact of hormones on our health. But by the mid-1970s, the scientific evidence surrounding HRT began to take on a kind of "seesaw" characteristic. Studies were cropping up linking the use of estrogen to an increased risk of cancer, first uterine cancer and then breast cancer. Then, in 1980, studies found that progestins could protect a woman's endometrium from cancer. Soon, combination estrogen/progestin HRT replaced estrogen-only HRT for women who still had their uteruses. By 1985, studies were showing that conventional HRT helped to protect against bone loss and maybe even heart disease.

Then, in 1989, *The New England Journal of Medicine* reported on a Swedish study that found a slight increase in the incidence of breast cancer among women who took estrogen, and twice that incidence in women who took estrogen and progestin therapy. And yet, in spite of these findings, in 1995 Prempro, the first all-in-one pill combination of Premarin and Provera was approved by the FDA. By 2001, more than 11 million women were using a Premarin product.

And then, in 2002, came scientific findings that were heard 'round the world. Early that year, both the HERS and its follow-up study, the HERS II, found an increased risk of heart attack, stroke, blood clots, and breast cancer in women using Prempro. By summer, the WHI study confirmed that it too had found an association between the use of Prempro and these risks. The news rocked the scientific and medical communities. The Premarin family of hormone products was, after all, the gold standard of replacement therapy. Within days, the Food and Drug Administration issued an order requiring all hormone products to carry a warning label. It seemed as if the death knell was being sounded for HRT. After nearly fifty years of valid scientific inquiry, how could this happen? To answer this question, we have to look back again.

A PARALLEL ROAD: NATURAL HORMONE THERAPY

During the 1980s and 1990s, the research on conventional HRT was really telling only half of the hormone story. Some scientists and researchers were actually taking another scientific road, a road that was going to revolutionize our thinking about hormones.

As far back as the 1940s and 1950s, European physicians were treating premenstrual syndrome (PMS) with natural, identical-to-human progesterone. In the United States, in contrast, women with PMS were being treated with oral contraceptives containing synthetic progestins, or with tranquilizers and antidepressants. But, in 1979, the first PMS patient in America was treated with natural progesterone replacement. The good news about the success of her treatment traveled fast, and over the next two years more than 500 women in the United States were treated with natural progesterone. Their treatment was highly successful. They did not experience the side effects associated with synthetic progestins, tranquilizers, and mood elevators.

By the mid-1980s, word had spread about the effectiveness of natural progesterone replacement, and scores of physicians and health-care practitioners across the country began using it to treat their patients with PMS. Hormonal imbalances were now being relieved with natural hormone replacement. But that was just the beginning of what we were going to learn about women and hormones from treating PMS with natural hormone replacement therapy.

The treatment of women with PMS was also revealing the highly individual way in which hormones function in a woman's body. Among women with PMS, there was a startling amount of variability, in both their symptoms and their responses to treatment. Some women had symptoms that occurred right before menstruation, whereas others had symptoms that occurred much earlier in their monthly cycle. There were women who had PMS every month, and there were those who had it every other month. There were even women who had PMS only at certain times of the year. And this variability from woman to woman was not restricted to symptoms alone. Some women's symptoms could be worsened by certain foods, or improved with lifestyle changes such as abstinence from alcohol or sugar. Some women responded to treatment with progesterone only, and some needed estrogen as well. Some women required only small dosages to relieve symptoms, whereas others needed much higher doses. Each woman, it seemed, had a hormonal constellation that was uniquely her own.

And then saliva testing, a new application of an existing technology, gave us a window into the body that set us on a course from which there would be no turning back. Saliva hormone-level tests showed that women produced different amounts of endogenous hormones. Saliva testing also confirmed that women who were given the same prescriptions for replacement hormones often responded in completely different ways. Not only did their baseline hormone levels play a role in how they responded, but there was also tremendous variability in how their bodies processed the hormones. Suddenly we had a whole new view of the behavior of hormones in the body. The same dosage of a hormone could produce different effects in the women taking it. And at the same time, different dosages could produce similar effects. In other words, one woman could take 25 milligrams of progesterone and another could take 400 milligrams, and their hormone levels would rise to a similar place. Or two women could each take 400 milligrams, and one woman's hormone levels would go off the chart while the other's level would be right within the expected range. Every woman had her own individual way of utilizing replacement hormones. This knowledge revolutionized the way doctors could prescribe hormone therapy not only for women with PMS but for perimenopausal and menopausal women as well.

Individualizing a woman's treatment with hormones that matched her own, in the lowest doses necessary to meet her body's needs, began to yield infinitely better results—the relief of symptoms was no longer compromised by side effects. Women who were using individualized natural therapy were feeling better than women on conventional, one-size-fits-all HRT. So what happened? Why haven't all women been receiving natural hormone replacement therapy in this manner?

PATENTS AND PROFITABILITY

Americans are among the healthiest people in the world. We owe this boon in great health largely to the discoveries and innovations of the pharmaceutical industry. Without them we certainly wouldn't be experiencing the quality of life or the increase in life expectancy we are enjoying. However, the success of the pharmaceutical industry is based on the patent process. Patents produce profits, and profits fund studies. Wyeth-Ayerst, for example, has held the patent on its Premarin family of formulations for decades, with prescription sales of over $2 billion per year. This is a wrinkle in the very fabric of scientific research. The industry that expands our knowledge about how drugs and medications work in the body can also place some limitations on it as well.

In a kind of good news/bad news conundrum, much of what we have learned about hormones has come from studying products like Premarin and Provera, because they have been the focus of most of the industry-sponsored scientific research. They are also the most widely prescribed. This research spawned our understanding of the true potential of hormone replacement. Unfortunately, over the years it has also placed limits on some important areas of hormone research and made it difficult to get funding for studies involving other forms of replacement hormones, such as natural hormones.

To date, HRT has been predominantly defined by studies that involve one-size-fits-all synthetic and animal-derived hormone preparations, which is why the importance of the Women's Health Initiative extends well beyond its findings. Government-funded and sponsored by the National Institutes of Health, the WHI showed us that the very products the industry had tested and deemed to be safe and protective against disease were in fact not without risk. This does not tell us that all hormone products are unsafe. It simply makes us more aware of the challenges involved in hormone replacement therapy.

You can think of it like this: Auto safety tests are conducted on an individual basis. If a particular model of car is found to be unsafe in a twenty-five-mile-per-hour collision, that doesn't necessarily mean that all cars are unsafe in the same situation. It may not even mean that the car would be unsafe in a ten- or fifteen-mile-per-hour impact. It simply means that that particular car could not stand up to that particular test challenge. Conversely, if a car is found to be safe in a twenty-five-mile-per-hour accident, this does not mean that all cars are therefore safe in the same circumstance. Nor does it mean that even a look-alike car can be assumed to be safe; each model needs to be tested individually for safety. Auto safety is determined car by car, challenge by challenge. Determining the safety and efficacy of hormone replacement therapy requires at least the same degree of scrutiny. We need more studies like WHI devoted to natural, identical-to-human hormone replacement.

Millions of women have used natural replacement hormones without suffering the side effects that come with conventional HRT. Because of this, the pharmaceutical industry is developing more and more natural hormone products. Natural hormones still cannot be patented; however, delivery systems can. New natural pharmaceutical hormone products in patch, gel, and spray forms are on the way. However, these products will still come in standardized dosages, which will not accommodate the unique hormonal needs of every woman. Excessive doses can cause side effects even when natural hormones are used.

Saliva testing has taught us that women can respond to infinitely smaller doses of replacement hormones than was previously believed—as much as a twentieth of what is commonly prescribed. Individualized, natural therapy allows a physician to tailor hormone therapy specifically to his or her patient's needs, in the lowest dose necessary, and to monitor her response.

WHAT ABOUT THE BREAST CANCER RISK?

Breast cancer is the biggest concern women have when they are considering hormone replacement. In fact, it is the number-one reason women decide against HRT. We believe that, in too many cases, the quality of women's lives is being compromised because they are afraid they will get cancer if they take replacement hormones. Yes, there is some evidence to suggest that hormones can play a role in breast cancer, but it is not a matter of "take hormones—get breast cancer." In fact, statistics show that 90 percent of the postmenopausal women who develop breast cancer have never taken HRT. There are many other culprits suspected of causing breast cancer in women, among them exposure to radiation, toxic chemicals, pollution, and viruses. All of these factors can cause the damage to DNA (the cells' genetic blueprints) that leads to cancer. Genetics is another factor. And remember, the average woman's risk of both heart disease and osteoporosis far exceeds her risk of developing breast cancer. In fact, even though the incidence of breast cancer is unacceptably high, most women do not develop it.

In recent years, there has been a reevaluation of the role hormone replacement plays not only in breast cancer but in other cancers as well. There is a substantial amount of scientific literature now that suggests we really don't know for certain that HRT does increase a woman's risk of cancer. Some of the latest research suggests that breast-cancer patients may not have to forgo the benefits of hormone replacement. For instance, a study done in Denmark demonstrated that there may even be some benefit to breast-cancer patients who take HRT. Their findings showed that there was no increase in the rate of breast-cancer recurrence in the women who used replacement hormones. Moreover, the women who were on HRT tended to survive longer.

Historically, oncologists and other physicians have believed that breast-cancer patients should not take hormone replacement therapy because the hormones would stimulate tumor growth. Yes, tumors can grow because hormones stimulate them. And studies have shown that unregulated, uncontrolled levels of estrogen may indeed contribute to breast-tumor growth. But this is not the whole picture. We are finding that it may not be the estrogen replacement itself that increases cancer risk, but the way in which it has traditionally been administered—by itself, without the protection of progesterone, and in doses that may be too high. One very important area of research today concerns the role that progesterone plays in protecting women from breast cancer.

In the body, during the luteal phase of a woman's menstrual cycle—when ovulation occurs and progesterone levels are very high—there is a distinct slowing down of estrogenic activity in the breast (see The Estrogen-Progesterone Pas de Deux in Chapter 3). This is similar to what happens in the endometrium as well. Progesterone has been shown to protect the endometrium and has been prescribed in conjunction with estrogen for that purpose. Of course, more studies are needed to validate this hypothesis; however, the slowing down of estrogenic activity in the breast when progesterone is present suggests that natural progesterone replacement may indeed be breast-protective. Interestingly, in both the HERS II and the WHI, the findings of an increased risk of breast cancer were associated with the use of synthetic progestin, not natural progesterone.

Play It Again—The Estrogen-Progesterone Pas de Deux

Statistics show that the incidence of breast cancer begins to go up when women enter their forties. This is about the same time that progesterone production begins to decline. During the previous twenty-five years of their lives—the years when most women are at their healthiest—they were producing proportionate amounts of both estrogen and progesterone each month. Once production of progesterone begins to drop off, there is a rise in the rate not only of breast cancer but also of uterine cancer, endometrial hyperplasia (an abnormal increase in the cells of the lining of the uterus), uterine fibroids, and fibrocystic breasts. All of these problems can be attributed to uncontrolled cell proliferation—the kind of cell growth that unopposed estrogen (that is, estrogen acting in the absence of the protective effects of progesterone) is most responsible for.

If we take a look at the many ways that progesterone works in the body, there are a number of reasons why it might be considered a cancer protective. Studies show that progesterone plays a role in the prevention of uterine cancer and possibly even breast cancer. Remember, progesterone actually decreases estrogen's activity by down-regulating estrogen receptors and blocking estrogen-stimulated cell growth (see page 31). Progesterone also boosts the activity of a type of white blood cells called *natural killer cells*. These are one of your immune system's first lines of defense against cancers of all types. Estrogens, in contrast, actually depress natural-killer-cell activity. We know from one study of women who underwent breast-cancer surgery that women who had progesterone in their bloodstreams (because they were in the second half of their menstrual cycles) at the time of the surgery were more likely to be alive fifteen years later than women who did not. No studies have been done yet to verify whether those same results would hold true with replacement progesterone, but it certainly seems to be an area that merits further investigation.

In animal studies of estrogen's role in cancer, it has been found that complementing estrogen with adequate amounts of progesterone dramatically reduces the incidence of some cancers. This suggests that if you take estrogen and progesterone together—the way they occur naturally in the body—the development of cancer may be less likely. In this way, science is showing us that it may not be the replacement hormones themselves but taking overdoses of individual hormones that increases the cancer risk. In other words, the problem may be the unregulated, uncontrolled activity of one hormone without the regulating, buffering action of its partners to balance it.

Evaluating the Data on HRT and Cancer

There is a great deal of data suggesting that estrogen replacement therapy can provide many different benefits to women as they age. And there is accumulating evidence that now suggests that progesterone is helpful in preventing most of estrogen's potentially negative effects. This presents a strong case for using both hormones together in any type of hormone replacement program.

Of course, no one should make general statements about cancer. Every woman is an individual, and her life and her body are unique. Whether a woman who is considered to be at high risk for breast cancer or is a breast-cancer survivor should consider HRT is something that only she can decide, in consultation with her doctor.

There are some researchers in the field of endocrinology and hormone replacement who believe that progesterone is a neutral hormone and plays no role at all in either causing cancer or protecting against it. There are others who believe that progesterone also stimulates breast tissue and that women who have a history of breast cancer should not use it. This topic is extremely controversial. We cannot say that using progesterone with estrogen will completely eliminate all cancer risk. All we can do is offer information. We need more studies to examine the role that progesterone plays in protecting against cancer and preventing it. Unfortunately, getting the results of those studies could take another twenty years or more. If you are considering HRT and you have questions about its relationship to cancer, being aware of the scientific research that is already available will help you make an informed decision.

The conventional medical approach to hormone replacement therapy has been based on a one-size-fits-all principle. That means that everyone who is a candidate for hormone replacement gets basically the same prescription. Not surprisingly, this approach has not yielded the results the medical community was after. What is wrong with this picture? It's really quite simple. There is one very spectacular omission in this type of treatment—the individuality of every woman's hormonal needs. What works for one woman does not necessarily work for another. The one-size-fits-all method is an outmoded and ineffective way to prescribe replacement hormones.

As humans, we are very similar: We each have a heart, a brain, lungs, kidneys, skin, and a skeletal system. But as an individual, each of us also is unique. For instance, some of us develop muscle very quickly when we exercise; others do not. Some of us seem to have endless energy; others need eight hours of sleep every night just to function. We have all known some people who can eat just about anything and not gain weight, and others who say, "If I even look at a candy bar, I gain five pounds." And, most likely, we have all known someone who needs twice as much pain medication as everyone else when he or she goes to the dentist. Individuality abounds. And individual variation abounds in hormone replacement therapy as well. In the next chapter, we will look at what needs to be changed about the way we prescribe and use HRT.

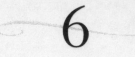

CHANGING THE STATUS QUO

When a woman enters menopause and her body begins to change, she is likely to make an appointment with her doctor to find out whether she is actually beginning to go through "the change." That's exactly what Francine did.

Francine was a 49-year-old real estate agent who had always taken very good care of herself. She ate a well-balanced, low-fat diet, supplemented with vitamins and minerals, and exercised regularly. But in spite of her healthy approach to life, Francine's occasional hot flashes were gradually in- tensifying and becoming more frequent. A person who prided herself on her sharp wit and her keen sense of humor, Francine also noticed that she was feeling "the blues" more often, and most of the time for no apparent reason. Francine decided to discuss her concerns with her doctor.

During her doctor appointment, Francine admitted that, along with her other symptoms, she was also having difficulty remembering things. At first she had attributed it to having too much on her mind, but all too often now she was forgetting where she put things or losing her thoughts right in the middle of a sentence. Francine's doctor listened intently and then explained to her that her symptoms, combined with her age and the fact that her cycles seemed to be waning, led him to believe that she was entering menopause and that her estrogen level was low.

Francine's doctor gave her a prescription for 0.625 milligrams of Premarin and 2.5 milligrams of Provera, the most commonly prescribed form of hormone replacement therapy. Within a week, Francine was on the phone with her doctor, reporting that her symptoms seemed worse. In addition, her breasts were very tender, she felt bloated all the time, and she could swear she was gaining weight. She didn't understand what was happening.

Unfortunately, all too often this is what a woman experiences when she first begins to have hormonal difficulties. Francine's menopausal symptoms were actually made worse by the treatment her doctor prescribed, because her prescription for Premarin was giving her more estrogen than she needed. In fact, Francine didn't need estrogen at all—she really needed only progesterone. To further complicate matters, she was not responding well to the Provera, which is a a synthetic form of progesterone.

As many as 80 percent of doctors who prescribe hormone replacement therapy still rely on empirical observation—that is, what they see—to determine whether a woman is menopausal and, if she is, what type of treatment to give her. But as we will see in this chapter, there is much, much more to hormone replacement than meets the eye.

OUT WITH THE OLD, IN WITH THE NEW

Your hormones are constantly responding to the ever-changing needs of your system. How old you are, how tall you are, and how much you weigh all have an impact on your hormonal landscape. Your overall state of health, your lifestyle, and even your state of mind all play a role in your hormonal profile as well. Your hormonal needs are unique to you.

If you take the replacement hormones that you need, in the amounts that are right for you, you will respond to them in a positive way. If, on the other hand, you take replacement hormones you do *not* need, or if you take more of a given hormone than is appropriate for you, any of a whole host of reactions can occur. You may gain weight, your breasts might swell and become uncomfortably tender, your blood pressure may go up, or you might start having random menstrual cycles at a time when you thought having your period was behind you. Or you may have no specific tangible symptoms but know that you just don't feel quite right. The individuality of how you absorb hormones, and how your body processes and eliminates them when their job is done, all contribute to how you feel and the way your body functions.

According to the *Physicians' Desk Reference* (PDR), a comprehensive resource that provides information on prescription medications, determining the correct dose of Estrace, a commonly prescribed form of replacement estrogen, is guided by "clinical response at the lowest dose in which symptoms are observable." This means the doctor has to determine what dose to give the patient by observing what happens to her symptoms. If the first dose tried alleviates the patient's symptoms, it is probably working. If her symptoms don't go away, the physician can try a higher dose—which might work, but, then again, might not.

We believe that instead of being based on a vague trial-and-error approach, a woman's HRT prescription should be determined on the basis of what her body actually needs. The solution for menopausal symptoms is not the same for all women. Some women need both estrogen and progesterone. Others need progesterone alone, especially in the early stages. For some women, testosterone or DHEA might be the answer. Still others need a combination of all four of these hormones.

Furthermore, in recent years, we have seen many innovations in the way women can take replacement hormones. They are now available in many different forms. First of all, there are synthetic hormones, animal-derived hormones, and natural, identical-to-human hormones. Second, replacement hormones come in tablet, capsule, cream, gel, patch, suppository, and implant forms. Does it matter what kind of hormone you take or what form it comes in? Yes, because each formula and each delivery system work differently in the body. Each of these variables counts as much as the others in determining the success or failure of your hormone replacement program.

Using the empirical method suggested in the PDR gives rise to many important questions. Simply observing an individual woman's symptoms does not help to determine which hormones are appropriate for her, nor can it tell her doctor what dosage to try first. To begin with, if you rely on observation alone, and a woman's symptoms do not go away when she is on HRT, how can you know whether the dosage is causing the problem? What if it is the wrong hormone? What if the delivery system isn't right? What if there is a problem with the sensitivity of the woman herself? Then, too, what if a woman has no menopausal symptoms but does have low hormone levels that put her at risk for osteoporosis and other degenerative diseases such as heart disease? How do you determine whether she needs replacement hormones? And if she is a candidate for hormone replacement, how would you determine how much to give her? Simply put, it is virtually impossible to know by observation alone how much of a hormone a woman needs or how much she is absorbing. And if a woman is taking a combination of hormones, just observing symptoms cannot tell you how the synergy of the hormones is affecting the outcome of her therapy.

Clearly, standard hormone replacement therapy, with its one-size-fits-all doses of synthetic or animal-derived hormones, cannot work for everyone. Consequently, even though researchers are heralding a brave new world of longevity and fitness for women, and are telling us that hormones may be the key, many women are not enjoying the benefits of hormone replacement, including many women who are currently on HRT.

Replacement hormones should do what your own hormones do naturally. The goal of a hormone replacement program, after all, is for you to feel as vital and healthy as you did when your own hormones were at their optimum levels. In order to accomplish this, you have to take into consideration not only the individuality of your own hormonal profile but all the complexities of the replacement hormones as well. In any hormone replacement program, you play a role and so do the hormones. For hormone replacement therapy to reach its full potential and fulfill its promise, the medical community is going to have to change the way it thinks. Individualizing and monitoring natural hormone replacement is the future of HRT.

UNDERSTANDING REPLACEMENT HORMONES

The best way to take replacement hormones is to take the ones that most closely resemble the ones your body makes for itself, in the amounts your body needs to function optimally—like it did when you were in your hormonal peak of health. The kind of hormone you take is as important as how much. All replacement hormones are not created equal. There are natural hormones, and there are synthetic and animal-derived hormones. And the differences between them can make a significant difference between whether you feel terrific or terrible on HRT.

Most of the hormone products commonly prescribed today are either synthetic or animal-derived. They are manufactured and marketed by major pharmaceutical companies and include all of the different brands of oral contraceptives as well as the commonly prescribed Premarin and Provera. All of them are chemically similar to your own hormones but not an exact match.

Natural replacement hormones also are prescription medications. They are highly purified pharmaceutical chemicals originally derived from wild yams and soybeans. They are produced by leading pharmaceutical companies and are regulated by the Food and Drug Administration. Many people believe that these hormones are called *natural* because they come from plants. But even though they do originate from plants, they are not plant or herbal extracts. They have to be converted in a laboratory into actual hormones. Once they have been through this process, they have a molecular structure that is identical to that of the sex steroid hormones your body makes for itself. So the term *natural* refers to their molecular structure, not to their source. Natural hormones are identical to your own hormones and natural to your body. That is why they are called natural hormones.

Lock and Key

Why does it matter whether replacement hormones are an identical match or just similar to your body's hormones? It matters most when a hormone binds with its receptor. Hormones are meant to fit perfectly with their receptors. Remember the key to that new Toyota Camry we talked about in Chapter 2? Because of the way a hormone has to fit with its receptor, its molecular structure is very important to the way it works in your body.

When a molecule of natural replacement progesterone travels through your bloodstream and binds with a progesterone receptor, the fit is the same as if the progesterone had been created in your own body—like they were made for each other. On the other hand, a molecule of synthetic progestin such as Provera, with a chemical structure only slightly different from that of progesterone, in actuality is a completely different molecule. The receptor can be fooled by it, but it doesn't fit quite right. It's a bit like putting on a shoe that is too small or too large, too narrow or too wide. You can get by with it, but if you wear it all day, it won't feel right. It may even cause you some very real discomfort. Similarly, if an altered form of a hormone is introduced into your body, instead of being useful for PMS or menopause symptoms, it can actually make them worse.

Many women experience side effects from synthetic or animal-derived hormones. These include weight gain; increased blood pressure; swollen, tender breasts; bloating; and feelings of anger, irritability, or depression. When women have their prescriptions changed to natural hormones, they get almost immediate relief. Natural replacement hormones fit with your hormone receptors like they are supposed to.

The structure of a replacement hormone is also important when the hormone has completed its job at the receptor site and the time has come for the hormone to be metabolized (broken down). The enzymes that metabolize hormones are very discerning. If they do not recognize a hormone molecule as one they are supposed to work on, they will pass it by. This can create problems because the hormone then sits on the receptor site longer than it should.

Another example we can look at is ethinyl estradiol (a synthetic form of estrogen used in oral contraceptives). Chemically, it is very similar to natural estradiol. However, the slight difference between these two molecules results in ethinyl estradiol being as much as a thousand times more potent than natural estradiol. During the 1940s, the alteration of estradiol into an oral contraceptive was one of the first manipulations of a natural hormone into a patented chemical. For birth control, ethinyl estradiol can be very effective, but for relief of menopausal symptoms it is much too strong.

Premarin, the number-one-prescribed type of replacement estrogen in the world, is an animal-derived form of estrogen. It contains equilin, or estrogen derived from the urine of horses. It too is similar in structure to human estradiol, but it is not a perfect match. Consequently, when equilin binds to an estradiol receptor in a woman's body, it does not fit exactly. It also prevents her own estradiol molecules from binding with their receptors. Further, because a woman's enzymes are designed to metabolize her own estrogens, they do an inefficient job of metabolizing equilin. Therefore, equilin stays on the receptor longer than natural estradiol does. A woman's own estradiol molecules are cleared from her system within hours. Equilin, on the other hand, has been shown to remain in the body for up to *thirteen weeks*. This can lead to overstimulation of the receptors and possible side effects. And when the equilin finally is metabolized, it results in the production of a metabolite that is considerably more potent than the equilin itself in its effects on the lining of the uterus. Thus, even though the structural differences between synthetic, animal-derived, and natural hormone replacement molecules are slight, when it comes to the influence they have on receptors—and on you—they do, in reality, make a big difference.

Synthetic and animal-derived hormones also generally come in standard, one-size-fits-all doses. They are made with additives and tablet coatings that can cause side effects of their own, including burning in the urinary tract, allergies, and joint aches and pains. Now, these differences do not mean that synthetic and animal-derived hormones cannot be effective, but they do help to explain why so many women have difficulty taking conventional HRT.

Most of the information we have on the benefits of HRT comes from studies done on Premarin and Provera. And some women do just fine taking them. But these forms of HRT are no longer alone on the playing field. Many pharmaceutical companies are now developing natural hormone replacement products because they have recognized their benefits over synthetics.

Even though we have known for a long time how beneficial estrogen replacement is, science has also known that taking estrogen alone can increase the risk of endometrial cancer. The solution then became to prescribe estrogen with a progestin like Provera in the hope that it would offer endometrial protection. However, thanks to the Postmenopausal Estrogen/Progestin Interventions (PEPI) study (see page 57), we now understand that taking natural replacement progesterone with estrogen not only provides women with protection against endometrial cancer but also benefits their lipid profile (the amounts and relative proportions of different types of fats and cholesterol in the blood) more than synthetic progestin. This is beneficial to the heart. In this study, 900 women were given various combinations of estrogen and progestin, and estrogen and natural progesterone. The study found that when estrogen was combined with the natural progesterone, it provided better cardiovascular protection than when it was combined with synthetic progestin. Once again we see that studies suggest hormone replacement therapy offers us the promise of a longer, happier, healthier, and more vital life, and that taking replacement hormones in the way that most closely resembles nature's own design is the best way to take them.

A Little Goes a Long Way

Your hormones are constantly building up, breaking down, and then rebuilding every aspect of you. They stimulate growth, regulate it, and then call a halt to it. In order to do all this, they work together, synchronistically. We have seen how taking replacement hormones can have a powerful influence on how (and when) you age. But we have also seen that too much of a hormone can be bad for you.

We measure hormones in an array of denominations and amounts that can boggle the imagination. When we measure levels of progesterone and cortisol, for example, we measure them in nanograms per milliliter (abbreviated ng/ml) of either blood or saliva. A nanogram is one-billionth of a gram (or $\frac{1}{28,000,000,000}$ ounce); a milliliter is the equivalent of $\frac{1}{5}$ teaspoon. Looking for something in nanograms is like looking for one specific person somewhere in the entire population of China—it gives new meaning to that old adage "like trying to find a needle in a haystack." Measuring your levels of estradiol, testosterone, or DHEA is even more of a challenge. These hormones are measured in picograms per milliliter (pg/ml). A picogram is one-*trillionth* of a gram. That's something like looking for one specific dollar bill somewhere in the entire 2.1-trillion-dollar budget of the United States.

Whether you are measuring hormones in nanograms or picograms per milliliter, the quantity of hormone in your blood amounts to something like a pinch of salt in an Olympic-size swimming pool. These numbers are quite astounding, aren't they? And so is the power of a molecule that can be effective at that level of concentration. When you think about your hormones in measurements this small, it makes you stop and wonder for a moment, if it takes so little of a hormone to do its job, how much is too much? How much is too little? Just how much does it take to put them out of balance? The answers to these questions are at the very heart of the hormone replacement dilemma.

If you are taking replacement hormones, you are increasing the amount of hormone you have circulating in your system. Because your hormones are all interrelated, taking one replacement hormone can affect the balance of your other hormones. It is very important to know what you have on hand before you start adding anything. Therefore, a crucial step in deciding if HRT is right for you is finding out what your own hormone levels are. And the way to do that is the subject of the next chapter.

7

HOW DO I KNOW IF HRT
IS RIGHT FOR ME?

The only way you can know for sure whether you need replacement hormones is to test your hormone levels. Knowing your hormone levels is as important as knowing your cholesterol level, your blood-sugar level, and your blood pressure. The only way to accurately determine if you are a candidate for HRT is to first find out what's going on with the hormones you have.

Hormone-level testing isn't a new concept. It has been a standard practice to measure thyroid-hormone and blood-sugar levels for years. And while it is not as routinely done, measurement of sex steroid hormone levels is possible as well. Physicians who do hormone testing have traditionally used blood tests to determine hormone levels. But blood tests have some limitations, as we will see in this chapter.

OLD, OUTMODED STANDARDS HAVE TO GO

When Beverly, a married 48-year-old high-school teacher with two grown children, suddenly started skipping periods, it gave her quite a start. The first two times it happened, she thought she might be pregnant. For most of her life, Beverly's cycles had been reliable and relatively stress-free. In fact, she joked that she could practically set her watch by them. But after she skipped the first one, missed cycles started occurring every few months, and it was unsettling to her.

In addition to skipping periods, Beverly also noticed that she was having dramatic fluctuations in her energy level. One day she would feel like she could climb any mountain, and then the next day she would feel tired enough to stay in bed all day. Some nights she would fall into bed and drop right off to sleep, and others she felt like getting up and spring-cleaning the entire house. She also noticed that her hair and skin felt dry, and there seemed to be more and more of her hair in her hairbrush and on the bathroom floor. And it wasn't just her hair and skin that seemed to be changing. Sometimes, when she was making love with her husband, her vaginal tissues were dry and she was uncomfortable. Even though she thought she was too young to be going through menopause, her symptoms were disconcerting to her, so she made a doctor's appointment.

Beverly's doctor did not seem alarmed by any of her complaints. He suspected she might be in the early stages of menopause, so he ordered a blood test to determine what her FSH and LH levels were. The results showed her to be in the normal range for a woman still having menstrual cycles. Her doctor told Beverly that her hormone levels were "fine," that she was not in menopause yet, and that she did not need any hormone replacement.

This is a very common experience for women who are in perimenopause or the early stages of menopause. This is because one of the most common blood tests that physicians use to determine whether a woman is in menopause does not even test her level of estrogen or any of the other sex steroid hormones. Rather, it tests for levels of two other hormones: follicle-stimulating hormone (FSH) and luteinizing hormone (LH) (see A Closer Look at the Menstrual Cycle, page 85).

Unfortunately, an FSH/LH test is not an accurate way to determine whether a woman is in menopause. There are too many ways to misinterpret the test results. While a woman is in transition from regular menstrual cycling to menopause, an FSH/LH test cannot reflect everything that is going on with her hormones. While it may reveal some of what is going on with her estrogen and progesterone levels, it does not give information about what is happening to her testosterone and DHEA.

A CLOSER LOOK AT THE MENSTRUAL CYCLE

⌐

Contrary to what many people believe, a woman's menstrual cycle is not controlled by hormones alone. The brain is involved, and so is the nervous system. The nerves of the hypothalamus (the part of the brain that regulates and controls appetite, body temperature, and many other vital bodily functions) and hormones work together. This is at least one of the reasons why stress, nervousness, and anxiety can affect a woman's menstrual cycle.

When you were about to enter puberty, a complex mechanism that involved your brain, your nervous system, and your ovaries signaled your body that it was time to begin menstruating. This mechanism is mysterious and powerful, and we still don't completely understand every aspect of it. But we do know that the time the process begins seems to be determined by body mass. In other words, when your body reaches a certain size, the mechanism is triggered. Then nerves connected to the hypothalamus signal for the release of a hormone called *gonadotropin-releasing hormone* (GnRH), which travels to your pituitary gland and stimulates the production of another hormone, *luteinizing hormone* (LH). LH is soon joined by yet another hormone, *follicle-stimulating hormone* (FSH), and a fluctuating nocturnal rise and fall of both hormones begins. Shortly after this happens, you enter puberty and have your first menstrual cycle.

The relationship between LH, FSH, and your sex steroid hormones is based on a complicated negative-feedback mechanism that involves your brain and your hormones. This feedback mechanism controls the production and release of your hormones through a complex system of checks and balances. For example, FSH stimulates the production of estrogen. When a certain level of estrogen production has been reached, estrogen then "turns around" and inhibits the release of FSH.

To better understand this feedback mechanism, let us look more closely at the mechanics of your monthly cycle. The first phase of the cycle, from day one (the day your period starts) until approximately day fourteen (or when ovulation occurs), is called the *follicular phase*. The second phase, from ovulation until you start your next period, is called the *luteal phase*. During the follicular phase, estrogen is on the rise because your hypothalamus is releasing FSH, which signals your ovaries to ripen one of their follicles (eggs). As the egg matures, estrogen production continues to rise and to stimulate the buildup of your uterine lining. When estrogen peaks, generally in the middle of your cycle, it stimulates the release of LH from your brain. LH signals for an increase in progesterone, which in turn tells your ovaries it is time to release the egg. You are now entering the second phase of the cycle, which is dominated by progesterone. If the egg is fertilized, progesterone production stays elevated. If it isn't, progesterone drops, prompting the beginning of menstruation, and the whole cycle begins again. In short, FSH stimulates the growth of the egg, which stimulates the rise in estrogen, which stimulates the production of LH, which stimulates the production of progesterone, and so on.

Obviously, FSH and LH are major players in your menstrual cycles. As you approach menopause, it actually takes them a while to get the message that things just aren't going to function in the same way anymore. When you reach menopause and your ovaries no longer make estrogen, your estrogen level naturally falls. In a kind of desperate attempt to signal your ovaries to produce more eggs, and therefore more estrogen, your brain can continue to stimulate the production of FSH and LH for quite some time. In fact, it is not unusual for FSH and LH levels to stay elevated during perimenopause and menopause.

And an FSH/LH test will reflect only what is happening at the time of the test.

Because FSH and LH rise and fall during a regular monthly cycle, if a woman has an FSH/LH test during a month when she ovulates, everything may appear to be normal when in fact her estrogen and progesterone levels are already in decline. Perimenopausal women in this situation, who actually need hormone replacement and could benefit greatly from it, frequently are sent home believing there is nothing amiss with their hormones.

On the other hand, if a woman has the test during a month when she has missed a period, her FSH and LH levels could be elevated as her body attempts to stimulate her ovaries to ovulate and produce the amount of estrogen and progesterone needed during a regular monthly cycle. Her doctor could interpret this to mean that she is in menopause. As a result, she might be given a prescription for replacement hormones that she doesn't need just yet. Or she might believe that because she is now in menopause, she can no longer get pregnant. But she may not have actually reached menopause yet. She could cycle again, and during that time, her levels of estrogen and progesterone could return to normal (and she could get pregnant). Thus, an FSH/LH test is simply not the best way to determine what is going on with a woman's changing hormone levels.

Beverly left her doctor's office with many of her questions about what was going on with her body unanswered. If everything was still working the way it always had, why was she feeling so different? In fact, Beverly actually had very low levels of progesterone and declining levels of estrogen. Had her doctor been able to tell her this, she could have received hormone replacement, her symptoms could have been alleviated, and she would have had a better understanding of what was actually happening to her.

An FSH/LH test is one of the tests doctors use to diagnose women they suspect might be entering menopause, but it is not the only one. Some doctors do use blood tests to actually test hormone levels. But blood tests measure the total hormone content of your blood. That means they measure both bound and bioavailable, or free, hormones (see page 30). Remember, bound hormones are ones that are a kind of circulating reservoir, being held in reserve. They are not biologically active. So a blood test that cannot differentiate between bound and free hormones gives you information that simply is not that useful.

Knowing your total hormone count is a little like knowing how much money you have in a certificate of deposit (CD) account at your bank. The money is there, which is reassuring, but you can't use it right away. Free hormones, on the other hand, are like cash in your pocket. Knowing your free-hormone levels is like knowing how much money you have to spend right now. To determine your blood levels of free hormones, more sophisticated testing must be performed, but it is not routinely done.

YOUR SPITTING IMAGE: SALIVA TESTING

Some of the most profound scientific discoveries in recent history have come about as a result of saliva research. For example, did you know that a crime-scene investigator could determine whether or not you were the person who sent a ransom note just by examining the saliva you left on the postage stamp? That's right. Your saliva holds a complete imprint of your DNA. But that's not all your saliva can reveal about you. A few drops of your saliva can reveal whether you have had too much to drink or have been using illegal drugs. It can also reveal whether you have been exposed to a particular virus or have a genetic predisposition for certain diseases. And, finally, a small saliva sample can give you and your doctor a very precise evaluation of your hormonal profile.

To fully understand the role hormones play in our lives, we must understand what actually happens to hormone levels in our body—what makes them go up, what makes them come down, and what happens to our health and behavior when they do. Saliva research facilitates the scientific investigation of hormones in ways never before possible. It provides a valuable window into the action of hormones and has given us a better understanding of the hormonal differences among individuals. This has helped to further our knowledge of the interplay between our daily lives and habits and our hormonal balance and ratios. As a result, we now know not only that our hormones influence us but also that we have an effect on our hormones—sometimes by the very way we choose to live our lives.

Salivary hormone-level testing is changing the face of hormone replacement therapy. As it turns out, it is quite easy to measure free-hormone levels in saliva. This is because bioavailable hormone molecules easily enter the saliva through the cells of the salivary glands, whereas bound hormones do not. When you test for hormone levels in saliva, you get an accurate accounting of the free hormones that are circulating throughout your body and interacting with your hormone receptors. You know just what your hormones are doing for you, right now. We believe this is the best way to test for hormone levels.

In general, the level of free hormones in the blood is only about 1 to 2 percent of the total blood-hormone level. So if you look at a standard blood test for estrogen, you can only estimate the level of free estrogen. For example, Susie's blood estrogen test showed her *total* estradiol level to be about 320 pg/ml. But saliva testing showed her estradiol measurement, at its highest level, to be 3.8 pg/ml. This tells us exactly what Susie's *free*-hormone level is—what is active in Susie's body and working for her.

Another important difference between testing hormone levels in blood and in saliva has to do with the time of day you take the test. Most often, you need an office or lab appointment to have a blood test done. Even if a clinic has a walk-in policy, you are subject to the clinic's scheduling requirements, and you have to arrange your own schedule to get there. It can be difficult to make the same arrangements every time you have your hormone levels tested. Thus, blood testing for hormone levels often ends up being done somewhat randomly, at a different time of day every time you test. Can that affect the outcome of the test? Yes, it can.

Some women refer to themselves as "morning people." Others say they function better at night. And that can have a lot to do with your hormones. Hormone levels rise and fall throughout the day in a rhythmic pattern called *diurnal variation*. Your levels of DHEA, testosterone, and cortisol—the hormones that get you up and going—are all naturally higher in the morning than later in the day. Figure 7.1 illustrates the normal daily variation in testosterone levels over the course of a day.

We believe that diurnal variation is an important factor in testing hormone levels. Because the result of a hormone level test can be affected by the time of day you take the test, two readings of the same hormone can be different simply because you took the tests at different hours of the day. For example, Marge had a blood test for her testosterone level performed at three o'clock in the afternoon. Her blood test result showed that her total testosterone level was 150 pg/ml. Marge is 52 years old, and, according to her blood test, her testosterone level was low for her age. However, when Marge tested the free-testosterone levels in her saliva at eight o'clock in the morning, and then again at three in the afternoon, her test results told a different story. The saliva test results showed that Marge had 28 pg/ml of free testosterone in the morning and 15 pg/ml of free testosterone in the afternoon. This demonstrates normal diurnal variation, in fact, and normal levels of testosterone for a fifty-two-year-old woman. Had Marge been given a prescription for testosterone on the basis of her blood test, it could have elevated her free testosterone to a level that was too high.

Saliva testing is done in the privacy and comfort of your own home—

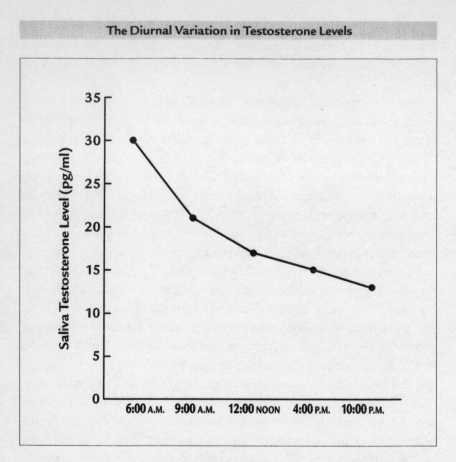

The Diurnal Variation in Testosterone Levels

FIGURE 7.1

Normal hormone levels vary according to not only the times of the month but also the time of day. Levels of DHEA, testosterone, and cortisol, for example, are all normally higher in the morning than later in the day. This phenomenon is called diurnal variation. *The graph above shows the normal variation in testosterone levels in women over the course of a day, as revealed by saliva testing.*

no appointment is necessary. This means you can easily do it at the same time of day every time you test. All you have to do is chew a piece of gum that is provided with the test, spit into a little plastic tube for a few moments, seal the tube up, and drop it in the mail to the testing lab. Saliva testing is reliable, economical, and stress-free—there are no needles involved. Within a few days you (and your doctor) know what your free-hormone levels are, and you can begin to make informed decisions about whether or not you need hormone replacement and, if you do, what doses are appropriate for you. You might say saliva testing gives you a "spitting image" of what your hormones are doing for you and what type of replacement hormones (if any) you need.

WHY HAVEN'T I HEARD ABOUT SALIVA TESTING?

When you consider that saliva testing is not only more convenient but also more accurate in assessing free-hormone levels, you may wonder why your doctor never recommended it—or, for that matter, why you have never even heard of it. It isn't because saliva testing is new. In fact, it has been used scientifically for over thirty years. However, until now, saliva testing has been used mainly in medical schools and research institutions.

Over the last fifteen years, the surge of interest in hormone replacement therapy has brought with it a growing demand, and a very real need, for this accurate method of testing hormone levels. In order to bring saliva testing to the public, every detail—from the type of container the sample is collected in to the time and fashion in which the sample is processed—had to be considered, in order to make sure this type of testing would be reliable. Thousands upon thousands of samples have been evaluated and interpreted according to gender, age, time of day, time of month, and time of life to establish normal ranges for different hormone levels for every age group. Table 7.1 shows normal saliva levels of progesterone and different estrogens. Table 7.2 lists normal levels of testosterone and DHEA. Normal levels of cortisol in women are in the range of 1.0 to 8.0 ng/ml in the morning and 0.1 to 1.0 ng/ml in the evening. Many years and a great deal of time, energy, and commitment have gone into the development and validation of saliva testing, and we now have a good scientific way to identify free-hormone levels. Instead of trying to guess what is going on with a woman's hormone levels, we now have actual physiologic evidence. We also have a way of knowing exactly how hormone replacement therapy affects her hormone levels. This can virtually put an end to the practice of over- and underdosing in hormone replacement therapy, which is so common in standard, one-size-fits-all HRT.

TABLE 7.1 NORMAL SALIVA LEVELS OF SEX STEROID HORMONES BY MENOPAUSE STATUS AND PHASE OF CYCLE IN WOMEN NOT TAKING HRT

This table reflects normal ranges of estradiol, estriol, estrone, and progesterone for pre-menopausal and postmenopausal women. Where appropriate, ranges for premenopausal women have been further broken down to represent normal levels for different periods within the menstrual cycle.

Hormone	Status	Normal Range
Estradiol	Premenopausal:	
	Follicular phase (first half of cycle)	0.5–5.0 pg/ml
	Midcycle (ovulation)	3.0–8.0 pg/ml
	Luteal phase (second half of cycle)	0.5–5.0 pg/ml
	Postmenopausal	<1.5 pg/ml
Estriol	Premenopausal	4.4–8.3 pg/ml
	Postmenopausal	3.0–11.8 pg/ml
Estrone	Premenopausal	2.6–5.4 pg/ml
	Postmenopausal	2.6–5.4 pg/ml
Progesterone	Premenopausal:	
	Follicular phase (first half of cycle)	<0.1 ng/ml
	Luteal phase (second half of cycle)	0.1–0.5 ng/ml
	Postmenopausal	<0.05 ng/ml

Further, salivary hormone testing gives us a map of what normal physiologic levels are with each passing decade of a woman's life. Because we now know how a woman's body ages hormonally, we have been able to develop target ranges of different hormones, or levels that are optimal for a woman's health. Saliva testing can tell us whether a woman is in her target range, so we can adjust the dosage of replacement hormones based not only on how she feels but also on how close she is to her target range. Finally, saliva testing has enabled us to better understand that every woman metabolizes and absorbs replacement hormones differently.

YOUR INDIVIDUAL HORMONAL PROFILE

Testing your hormone levels in saliva is like looking into a glass carriage. It lets you see exactly what is going on inside, right now. Saliva testing

TABLE 7.2 NORMAL SALIVA LEVELS OF TESTOSTERONE AND DHEA IN WOMEN

This table reflects normal ranges of testosterone and DHEA in women by age.

Age Range	Testosterone	DHEA
20–29	17–52 pg/ml	106–300 pg/ml
30–39	15–44 pg/ml	77–217 pg/ml
40–49	13–37 pg/ml	47–200 pg/ml
50–59	12–34 pg/ml	38–136 pg/ml
60–69	12–35 pg/ml	36–107 pg/ml
70–79	11–34 pg/ml	32–99 pg/ml
80 and over	——	33–90 pg/ml

lets you know where you are on your hormonal time line, and that helps you make conscious, informed decisions about the direction you want to take with hormone replacement therapy.

Saliva tests clearly demonstrate the diversity that exists in women's hormonal profiles and the importance of assessing each woman individually. Let us look at the saliva-hormone-test results of a group of women who are all about the same age. Table 7.3 shows the early-morning hormone levels of six different women as revealed through saliva testing. As you can see in the following pages, even though these women are close in age and are all experiencing some menopausal symptoms, the hormonal profile of each is uniquely her own.

Remember Lana? Lana, whose story appears in Chapter 3, was experiencing lots of symptoms—a lack of energy, mood swings, forgetfulness, insomnia, and a loss of sex drive. At 51, she was worried that she might need a little estrogen. Her saliva test revealed that her estrogen, at 0.8 pg/ml, is in fact low. But that's not all. Lana's progesterone and testosterone levels also are very low. This helps to explain many of her symptoms. So a simple prescription for Premarin and Provera might not do the trick for her.

Ellen is the same age as Lana, but, as you can see, saliva testing revealed that her hormone levels are very different from Lana's. Even though she has skipped a menstrual cycle or two, for the most part Ellen is still cycling. She does experience some PMS discomfort every month, but she does not have as many symptoms as Lana. Ellen's progesterone level is

TABLE 7.3 EARLY-MORNING HORMONE LEVELS OF SIX WOMEN				
	Estradiol	Progesterone	Testosterone	DHEA	Cortisol
Lana	0.8 pg/ml	0.06 ng/ml	18 pg/ml	110 pg/ml	4.7 ng/ml
Ellen	2.0 pg/ml	0.1 ng/ml	27 pg/ml	121 pg/ml	3.2 ng/ml
Deanna	2.3 pg/ml	0.4 ng/ml	36 pg/ml	143 pg/ml	2.8 ng/ml
Melanie	1.3 pg/ml	0.02 ng/ml	23 pg/ml	96 pg/ml	5.8 ng/ml
Annette	0.7 pg/ml	0.01 ng/ml	25 pg/ml	79 pg/ml	4.6 ng/ml
Veronique	0.6 pg/ml	0.01 ng/ml	26 pg/ml	87 pg/ml	3.5 ng/ml

low enough that it might be the culprit in her recurring PMS symptoms. On the other hand, her estradiol, DHEA, testosterone, and cortisol levels are all well within the normal range. Thus, Ellen would most likely benefit from some progesterone replacement.

Deanna, 46, is still having very regular menstrual cycles and feeling terrific. She is experiencing no menopausal symptoms whatsoever. And no wonder: Her hormone levels are all within the range you would expect to see in a woman her age.

Melanie is 47 and complaining of some typical perimenopausal symptoms. She feels like her moods change suddenly for no apparent reason, her hair is falling out in a way that frightens her, her cycles are completely unpredictable, and she feels like she is gaining weight around her tummy even though she has not changed her eating habits. Melanie's hormone levels are all very good, with the exception of her progesterone level, which is low enough to be wreaking havoc with how she feels. This is what commonly happens in perimenopause—progesterone is the first to decline. In Melanie's case, her test results indicate that she may not be ovulating any longer and that some progesterone would most likely be helpful. It is interesting to note that even though both Melanie and Ellen may be experiencing symptoms because of their low progesterone levels, none of their hormone levels is exactly the same.

Annette is the same age as Melanie, and she is complaining of many of the same symptoms. Plus, Annette is having drenching night sweats and hot flashes all day long. And, indeed, her test results show that Annette also has stopped ovulating, but in her case, estradiol is declining as quickly as progesterone. The rest of her hormones are right in line with what they should be during perimenopause.

Now let's meet Veronique, who is 52 years old and in menopause. Veronique feels great and seems to be breezing through her change without any outward signs or symptoms. Even though she feels terrific, when we compare Veronique's hormone levels to those of a woman who is still menstruating, we can see that they fall considerably below the more youthful range that used to afford her protection from heart disease and osteoporosis. If a woman has a family history of either of these "silent" diseases, this information can be very valuable. For Veronique, saliva testing offers inside information that her body is not yet telling her. Her hormones are no longer providing her with as much protection against degenerative disease as she might want.

SALIVA TESTING AND YOUR RESPONSE TO HRT

Saliva tests not only tell you what your free-hormone levels are but also help you effectively monitor the complex interactions and delicate relationships that hormones have with one another. Remember, when you are considering HRT, not only are your specific needs an important factor but so too is the unique and individual way you respond to replacement hormones. A saliva test can help you to determine how you are responding to your therapy by telling you how your hormone levels are being affected.

By compiling and evaluating the test results of thousands of patients, we have been able to define expected hormone-level ranges that reflect both normal, unsupplemented levels at various ages and levels achieved with various forms of supplemention. Expected ranges take into account the high degree of variability in hormonal profiles from woman to woman and give us some guiding parameters for the lower and upper ends of hormonal functionality. Patient studies have revealed that individuals with more youthful hormone levels have fewer menopausal symptoms and reduced malaise. Remember, your body has an innate knowledge of how much of each hormone it needs in circulation to function properly. If there is too much or too little of a given hormone, symptoms, side effects, and even disease can result. Using expected ranges to evaluate a woman's baseline hormone levels can help to determine which replacement hormone (or hormones) a woman may need to relieve symptoms. Then, once she begins hormone therapy, expected ranges provide a guide for monitoring how her body is responding to it. Keeping in mind that every woman metabolizes and utilizes replacement hormones in her own way, using a combination of expected hormone level ranges and an ongoing assessment of symptoms can help to determine whether a woman's levels have been sufficiently elevated or have reached the upper limit and are too high. It is important to remember that there is never a reason to take more of a hormone than you need. The expected ranges are guidelines that can help you to achieve an effective hormone replacement program that is designed especially for you, using the lowest possible doses.

Unfortunately, for women who are taking conventional HRT, saliva testing cannot reveal the entire impact of their therapy. Saliva hormone testing relies on unique identifiers such as antibodies in order to measure the level of a type of molecule precisely. Identifiers do not exist that can measure all of the equine (horse) estrogens in conventional HRT products such as Premarin or Prempro. We can measure the small amount of estradiol in the product and we can tell how high your estradiol and estrone levels are being raised, but this is a limited picture because of the numerous other ingredients in these products. Similarly, there are no identifiers for synthetic progestins, so hormone-level testing cannot monitor the effect of Provera. This is a significant drawback to synthetic progestin therapy when you understand the importance of monitoring a woman's response to HRT.

Assessing your hormonal profile with a saliva measurement is the best way to find out if you need hormone replacement. Once you clearly know where you stand hormonally and you are ready to make decisions about whether hormone replacement is right for you, you will be faced with yet another question: How much of a replacement hormone should you take? Saliva hormone-level monitoring tells you how you are responding to your HRT.

Let's look at Sharon and Marie Helene. They are different in many ways. Sharon is 52 and Marie Helene is 59. Their first saliva tests showed that they had identical estradiol levels, 0.6 pg/ml. Each was given an oral dose of 0.25 mg of estradiol to be taken twice a day. When Sharon and Marie Helene were retested, their new estradiol levels truly reflected their individual responses to therapy. Sharon's estradiol level was 0.9 pg/ml, which is low. The prescribed dose was clearly not enough for her. But it was just right for Marie Helene; it brought her estradiol level up to a desirable 2.3 pg/ml.

Given all the complexities of your endocrine system and the infinitesimal amount of a hormone that it takes to do its job, knowing what is right for you is the only rational way to take replacement hormones. One of the greatest challenges we are faced with in accomplishing this is determining the amount of hormone it takes to both relieve symptoms and provide the disease protection you enjoyed while you were still menstruating, and to do this without causing side effects. Because hormones are so powerful and every woman's response to them so different, it is important to have an HRT prescription filled by someone who understands all the nuances of hormone replacement and individualized therapy.

Not only is the dose of a replacement hormone important, but the delivery system (pill, cream or gel, patch) it comes in has an enormous impact on how it works in your body. Because of this, the pharmacist can play a significant role in the outcome of your hormone replacement therapy. When you know just what you need, and you take it in a way that has been formulated specifically for you, hormone restoration can be a very positive experience. In the next chapter, we will see how individualizing and monitoring hormone replacement is better medicine for women.

PHARMACY FOR THE
TWENTY-FIRST CENTURY

Most women today who have been given "one-size-fits-all" hormone prescriptions by their doctors take the prescription to a drugstore to have it filled. The pharmacist behind the counter fills the prescription from a container of premade, standard-dose pills. Unless there is an emergency, there is no interaction between the doctor and the pharmacist or between the pharmacist and the patient. This is a very fragmented, impersonal approach to medical care. Fortunately, this is not the only way you can have a hormone prescription filled.

If you are going to have a hormone replacement program that consists of a natural hormone prescription that is designed especially for you, you will have to have it formulated by a pharmacist who specializes in *compounding* (making prescriptions by hand) and *titrating* (individualizing the dosage). That means your prescriptions will be handmade especially for you.

Pharmacies that specialize in compounding and titrating medication exist all around the country. However, there is a great deal of diversity among them, not only in the ingredients they use but also in their methods of preparing prescriptions. For example, an important aspect of transdermal hormone creams, which deliver hormones through the skin, is the cream base that is used. Not all cream bases are the same. If you have a cream that tends to clump and remain on the surface of your skin without penetrating it effectively, then the hormone may not be able to pass freely through your skin and into your bloodstream. If the hormone is not getting into your body, then it isn't working for you. Using the most effective base is very important in formulating a transdermal cream.

Having your hormone replacement program formulated for you is best done by a pharmacy that specializes in women's health and hormone therapy. In this chapter, we will look at the key role the pharmacist plays in individualizing your therapy. In much the same way you would choose a doctor who specializes in the particular kind of medical condition you have, choosing a pharmacist to fill your HRT prescriptions is an important part of ensuring that you get the best possible care. It makes a difference in the success of your program to have a pharmacist who understands all the dynamics of the absorption and metabolism of replacement hormones working with you and your doctor.

TABLETS, PATCHES, CREAMS, AND MORE

A simple prescription for hormone replacement can actually provide a whole host of different effects. This is because prescriptions come as capsules, tablets, creams, gels, patches, and suppositories, and each form works differently in the body. Scientists refer to these methods of taking hormones as *delivery systems.* Some delivery systems act very quickly; others have a more sustained, even effect. In addition, when prescription hormones are metabolized, some of the metabolites that result may be helpful, but others may be harmful. Understanding the different ways in which metabolites can affect your therapy can help you determine whether what you experience is a side effect or a desired effect.

The particle size of a prescription hormone is also very important. To understand particle size, think of different types of sugar. Granulated sugar (ordinary table sugar) is relatively coarse; powdered (confectioners') sugar is very fine. The difference between the two is a difference in particle size—larger for granulated sugar, smaller for powdered sugar. Even though powdered sugar looks and feels very different from granulated sugar, it is still sugar. This same kind of particle size difference exists among replacement hormones. Micronized hormones have the smallest particle size—under 10 microns—which is just about as small as you can get. As a result, micronized hormones are the most easily dispersed in a prescription formula and the most easily absorbed.

When you think about all the variables involved in a simple prescription for hormones, who better to assist you in making decisions about it than the pharmacist? The pharmacist is the person who understands the synergy between hormones and the differences between all of the available dosages and delivery systems. All of these factors are important in determining how much of a replacement hormone you should take and when. By being actively involved in your hormone replacement therapy program, the pharmacist can help you and your doctor better understand how and why your hormones affect you the way they do.

Julia is 59 years old. Recently, she slipped and fell as she was getting into her car. It was not a terribly dramatic fall, but when the pain didn't let up after a few days Julia made an appointment to see her doctor. Julia's doctor x-rayed her foot, and, sure enough, there was a fracture. Because Julia was postmenopausal, her fracture indicated to her doctor that her bones might be weakening. He urged her to begin estrogen therapy and prescribed a 1-milligram oral tablet of Estrace to be taken daily.

Julia remembered reading somewhere that when you take medications sublingually—that is, place them under your tongue and allow them to dissolve rather than swallowing them whole—they work faster and are absorbed better. She had been frightened by her fall, and she was very worried about her bones. She wanted her hormones to start working right away, so, without telling her doctor, she started taking her Estrace tablet sublingually. Even though sublingual medications are taken by mouth, they work very differently than tablets and capsules. Sublinguals are absorbed directly into the bloodstream, bypassing the digestive system. Sublingual dosages are generally very low because so much of the hormone is absorbed and goes directly to work.

Almost immediately after Julia began placing her Estrace tablet under her tongue, she started having symptoms. She felt terrible, almost as if she were going through menopause all over again, only worse. Headaches, bloating, nausea, breast tenderness—it was awful. She called her doctor right away, and he ordered a saliva test to see if her dose was a little too high. He was shocked by her results. Her estradiol level was 61.4 pg/ml, almost sixty times higher than it should have been. Julia's doctor didn't understand how that could have happened, so he called a pharmacist who specialized in individualized hormone replacement for a consultation.

The pharmacist looked over Julia's patient history and then suggested that her doctor ask Julia how many times a day she was taking her prescription and whether she was taking it with food. As a long shot, the pharmacist then asked if Julia could be putting the tablet under her tongue. The pharmacist also expressed concern that Julia wasn't taking any progesterone with the estrogen and explained to her doctor all the reasons why he might want to consider incorporating it into her hormone replacement program. Julia's doctor agreed to test her progesterone level.

When Julia told her doctor she was taking only one Estrace tablet each day but that she was, indeed, putting it under her tongue, he explained to her that by taking the tablet that way she was absorbing too much of the hormone and the excess hormone was causing her discomfort. He told her to swallow the pills instead. Julia followed his instructions and her symptoms went away. When she had her estradiol level tested again, it was 1.8 pg/ml— right where it should be. At that time her doctor also tested her progesterone level, which was 0.03 ng/ml. He gave her a prescription for a 125-milligram capsule of natural progesterone twice a day.

As you can see from Julia's story, the involvement of a pharmacist who specializes in individualized hormone replacement therapy made a big difference in how well her hormone replacement program worked for her.

Now let us take a look at some of the delivery systems available for hormone replacement. Formulating an individualized program means choosing what works best for you. That means both what works best in your body and what you feel most comfortable using. By becoming familiar with how hormone delivery systems work, you will be able to make choices that you feel at ease with and that will be the most effective for you.

Suppositories

Suppositories were one of the earliest forms in which supplemental hormones were available, and they are still used today. They are hormone preparations designed to be inserted vaginally, and they can be very effective. If you are going to use a vaginal hormone suppository, there are a few things to consider. First of all, vaginal tissue provides a large area for absorption. Second, it allows the hormone to be absorbed directly into your bloodstream, avoiding the first-pass elimination, in which the hormones are either broken down and eliminated or bound with carrier proteins and deactivated as they pass through the liver.

With vaginal suppositories, the composition of the suppository base is a significant factor. Some bases enhance the absorption of the hormones; other diminish it. A polyethylene glycol (PEG) base suppository works very well because it is nonirritating and provides a consistent, even release of hormone into the bloodstream. A cocoa-butter base, on the other hand, retains the hormone longer. As we have mentioned, sex steroid hormones are fat-loving molecules. In other words, they are more drawn to fatty substances than they are to watery substances. So if you have a suppository with a cocoa-butter base, the hormone naturally gravitates toward the fat in the base, and less hormone will actually get absorbed into your system. If the only symptom you are trying to manage is vaginal dryness, then a cocoa-butter-based suppository might be just fine. If you have other symptoms that require a more rapid and consistent release into your system, then the PEG base would probably be better for you.

Another important consideration with suppositories is their melting point. A suppository has to melt in order for the hormone to be absorbed. If a suppository isn't melting, it isn't working.

Bonnie was using a vaginal progesterone suppository. Even though she was using it as directed, she wasn't getting any relief from her symptoms. A saliva test suggested she was not absorbing the hormones in the suppositories. When we tested one of her suppositories, we found that its melting point was over 120°F.

It is highly unlikely that Bonnie's—or anyone else's—body temperature would ever reach 120°F. Were she to continue using that particular form of suppository, it is not likely she would get any symptom relief.

Orals: Capsules and Tablets

Hormones that are administered orally, in tablets or capsules, have to go through your digestive system before they can actually go to work for you. In the process, they are subjected to first-pass elimination by your liver (see page 102). Thus, the amount of hormone that is left to circulate throughout your system and work for you is only about 10 percent of the dosage you started with. In order to compensate for what is lost in this process, oral hormone dosages are generally fairly high.

As tablets and capsules go through your digestive process, they are metabolized, which, naturally, provides more opportunities for the creation of metabolites. Metabolites can play an important role in how your hormones work for you. For example, some women who take 100-milligram progesterone capsules can experience drowsiness or a feeling of lightheadedness that is a little like being at happy hour. The drowsiness is caused by the progesterone metabolites that bind to GABA receptors in the brain (see page 41). These metabolites can be more potent than a barbiturate. Of course, not all women respond the same way. Some women can take a 200-milligram capsule and not feel sleepy at all. It depends on how their bodies metabolize the replacement hormones. When you are taking HRT—or any medication—it is important to discuss what you experience with your doctor and a pharmacist who specializes in individualized HRT. Drowsiness can be considered a side effect. However, if you need something to help calm you at night or relieve some anxiety, you might consider it a desired effect.

There are many different oral formulations of replacement hormones. In general, products that contain micronized hormones suspended in oil are the best because they are the most readily absorbed. Suspending micronized hormones in oil further improves their effectiveness because the long-chain fatty acids in the oil act synergistically with the hormone and increase its absorption.

Linda was 46 and perimenopausal. She suffered from PMS—food cravings, mood swings, fatigue, breast tenderness, and migraines. She was also beginning to experience hot flashes. Linda was taking 200 milligrams of oral micronized progesterone twice a day, which was managing her symptoms very well, but she was complaining that she felt sleepy all the time. For Linda, this was definitely not a desired effect. In fact, fatigue was one of the symptoms she was trying to eliminate.

When Linda's physician reviewed her saliva test results, he could clearly see she was absorbing too much of her progesterone, as her progesterone level was 2.1 ng/ml. Her doctor suggested she try a vaginal suppository, and she agreed. As soon as Linda started using the suppositories, her drowsiness was relieved. And she still enjoyed relief from all of her other PMS symptoms.

For most women with PMS, however, we have found that taking progesterone orally, in sustained-release form, generally works best. The effects last for ten to twelve hours. In Linda's case, her response to 400 milligrams of progesterone warranted a lower dose and a different delivery system. For Terry, on the other hand, a timed-release tablet worked very well.

Forty-two-year-old Terry also suffered from PMS. Almost like clockwork, in the middle of each month, Terry became depressed and irritable, bloated, and mentally "foggy." Her progesterone level was 0.03 ng/ml, which is the level you would see in a postmenopausal woman, not a woman in her early forties. A daily 300-milligram timed-release progesterone tablet worked wonders for Terry. Her progesterone level went up to 0.33 ng/ml, very good for a woman her age. Her PMS symptoms went away, and she felt more like herself all month long.

Carol, 50 years old and in menopause, was using a transdermal progesterone cream and was quite happy with the results she was getting. The only symptom it seemed unable to alleviate was her insomnia. When Carol tested her saliva progesterone level, it was 0.1 ng/ml—the low end of the range for her. Carol's doctor consulted a pharmacist trained in individualizing HRT about Carol's insomnia, and the pharmacist suggested a 150-milligram micronized-in-oil progesterone capsule twice a day. Once Carol started using oral progesterone, she began sleeping peacefully through the night. When she was retested, her progesterone level was up to 0.27 ng/ml, a much more optimal level for her.

One question many women who take oral hormone preparations frequently ask is whether they should take their hormones with or without food. It is a very good question. When taken orally, sex steroid hormones don't usually cause stomach upset, so in that respect it doesn't matter. However, taking them with food can increase their absorption by as much as two to five times. This is not an increase in how quickly you absorb the hormone, but in the amount of the hormone that actually gets into your system, which affects your hormone levels. This increased absorption can be enhanced even further by eating high-fat foods. Remember, hormones are fat-loving molecules.

If you are taking replacement estrogen, the effect of food on absorption can become very significant. The estrogens are particularly vulnerable to what is called *enterohepatic recirculation*. This means that, instead of being eliminated from your system once it has done its job, an estrogen molecule can circulate throughout your gastrointestinal tract and reenter your system as a free hormone again. For example, estriol has always been considered a weak estrogen because it does not bind very tightly to estrogen receptors. And when it does bind to the receptors, it doesn't stay there very long. In most cases, estriol is not strong enough to stimulate the buildup of the lining of your uterus. So it doesn't usually cause breakthrough bleeding. Breakthrough bleeding is irregular or prolonged bleeding due to continual sloughing of the uterine lining that can occur during the menstrual cycle if you take oral contraceptives. It can also occur if you no longer have menstrual cycles but are taking HRT. Estriol is generally not strong enough to cause breakthrough bleeding, nor is it generally strong enough to stimulate breast tissue, which can cause swelling and tenderness. However, if you take estriol continually and it is recirculated in your system as free estriol, instead of being eliminated, the constant stimulation of your receptors can bring on these symptoms. It is a cumulative effect.

Karen was a 51-year-old woman with a family history of breast cancer. She wanted to use estriol for her menopausal symptoms because she believed it was safer than estradiol. But soon after she started using it, she experienced some spotty bleeding. Her doctor decided to monitor Karen's saliva estriol levels throughout the day, and found that her baseline level in the morning was 7 pg/ml. This reflects what her hormone level is before supplementation. Right after she took her test, at about 9:00 A.M., Karen swallowed a 4-milligram estriol capsule. After a high-fat lunch consisting of pasta Alfredo with salad, French bread and butter, and crème brûlée for dessert, her estriol level went up to 75 pg/ml. After her dinner, which was another high-fat meal—cheese enchiladas, chicken tacos with guacamole and sour cream, and vanilla ice cream—Karen's estriol level went up to an even higher 100 pg/ml. Because Karen was taking her estriol with her meals every day, she was achieving much higher levels than desired.

If Karen had not monitored her saliva hormone levels, she would never have known this. Karen stopped taking her prescription at mealtime, her symptoms were relieved, and her estriol level returned to normal.

Laila requested estriol from her doctor because she had heard it was very effective for vaginal dryness. Her doctor prescribed 3 milligrams of estriol to be taken once a day. During the first month on her estriol prescription, Laila experienced intense breast swelling and tenderness. This suggested that her breast cells were being overstimulated. When Laila had her saliva estriol level tested, it was indeed up to 80 pg/ml. Laila's doctor changed her prescription to an estriol suppository, to be used only three times a week. After a month of using her new prescription, Laila retested her estriol level, and it was 25 pg/ml. She was no longer experiencing any breast tenderness, and her vaginal dryness was gone.

Laila's experience is a fairly common one because estriol suppositories are very popular for vaginal dryness. If you are using an estriol suppository, it is best to use it once a day for the first week or two, and then only two to three times a week. In that way you ensure that your estrogen receptors are not overstimulated, which can result in breakthrough bleeding and breast swelling.

Transdermals

Transdermals are creams, gels, and patches that are applied to your skin. They are very popular because they are so easy to use. More important, however, some transdermal preparations, like patches, mimic your own hormone-releasing patterns very closely and provide very even, constant hormone levels. When you use a transdermal patch, the patch functions like a reservoir of hormones so that they are delivered into your system gradually. Patches provide you with consistent hormone levels that can closely resemble your own.

When you use a transdermal cream or gel, the hormones are absorbed rapidly and efficiently. Transdermally applied hormones enter your system as free hormones, which means they can go to work right away. Because they do not go through a first-pass elimination by your liver, dosages of transdermals can be lower than those of other delivery systems—as much as ten times lower than oral dosages. This is a significant decrease in the amount of hormone that a woman needs to use in order to enjoy all the benefits of HRT.

We conducted a study on the use of a transdermal progesterone cream involving thirty women who had postmenopausal symptoms including night sweats, hot flashes, and irritability. The women were divided into three groups of ten. The first group received a placebo (a cream that contained no hormone); the second received a cream containing a minimal dose of 5 milligrams of progesterone per ounce; and the third group received a cream containing 450 milligrams of progesterone per ounce. The study lasted for sixty days. All of the women who participated had baseline blood and saliva measurements of their progesterone levels taken before the study began and then had their levels monitored using blood and saliva samples during the study.

The women using the placebo cream experienced no changes in progesterone hormone levels and no relief of symptoms. In the women using the lower dose cream, there were only slightly measurable effects in saliva and only minimal relief of symptoms. Women taking the higher dose cream showed a very measurable effect on saliva progesterone levels and substantial symptom relief. Interestingly, the effect on their blood progesterone levels was also measurable, though not equal to that seen in saliva.

Here's another way of looking at those results: 25 milligrams of progesterone, the amount generally delivered in one-half teaspoon of cream containing 450 milligrams per ounce, markedly increases saliva levels of progesterone. And even though it also raises blood levels, most doctors who use blood testing would not see it as a very substantial elevation. A health-care practitioner familiar only with blood testing might therefore conclude that transdermal progesterone cream is poorly absorbed. The patient, on the other hand, could be feeling a great deal of symptom relief—her fibrocystic breasts might have improved, her mood might be better, and her hot flashes might have subsided. Based on her blood test, her doctor might believe her results are a placebo effect. This can be confusing to her and wouldn't seem to explain how she is feeling. The saliva hormone level does, however, more accurately reflect the true hormone-level rise. It demonstrates that patients can get symptom relief with small doses of hormone delivered transdermally. And this marked increase in saliva hormone level is not unique to progesterone; the same results can be expected when estradiol, testosterone, or DHEA is delivered transdermally.

Why would a doctor not conclude that the cream is working if he or she can see that a woman's symptoms were alleviated? Unfortunately, many doctors are not yet familiar with the use of natural hormones like progesterone, or with transdermal hormone creams, so they are somewhat skeptical about their use. At the same time, many doctors are comfortable relying on the tests they are the most familiar with. If these tests tell them the cream is not working, they may believe the test more than the patient and conclude that any relief she is experiencing is due to a placebo effect, even though it isn't.

Sarah was taking a 1-milligram Estrace tablet and a 100-milligram oral micronized progesterone tablet daily. Her saliva levels of both estradiol and progesterone suggested that these doses were too high for her. Sarah's doctor reduced her Estrace dosage to 0.25 mg of estradiol twice a day (half the dose she had been taking). He also changed her progesterone dose to one-eighth teaspoon of 2 percent progesterone cream, to be used morning and evening— considerably less than half of what she had been using.

Transdermal creams and patches have made it possible to use substantially lower doses of replacement hormones to achieve the same effect as higher doses of oral preparations. This is amply demonstrated by the medical community's rapid adoption of low-dose pharmaceutical patches, and it marks a revolutionary change in HRT. More important, new scientific literature demonstrates that lower doses of natural hormones, taken transdermally, do indeed provide bone protection and have a positive effect on cholesterol, helping to keep HDL ("good") cholesterol high and LDL ("bad") cholesterol low. That means that, even with minimal doses, a woman will receive the maximum benefit from her hormone replacement program. Many pharmaceutical companies are now creating lower dose patches.

When it comes to the absorption of transdermals, another consideration is where you apply them. You can apply them to your abdomen, thigh, or shoulder, or even rotate the sites. We conducted a study on the application sites of transdermals. It appears that the best absorption may actually be through the hands. Serendipitously, in one of the experiments, we had someone wearing latex gloves apply the hormone cream to the patients so that the patients wouldn't get any on their hands. When we tested the patients' levels, we found that their absorption was lower than when they had applied the hormone cream themselves using their hands. Further studies are needed to better evaluate application sites.

It is important to remember that it is possible to transfer transdermal hormones to another person, such as a child or a friend, or even your family pet. It's best to wash your hands immediately after applying a transdermal hormone preparation to avoid this. If you apply hormone cream, jump right into bed, and snuggle up to your partner, some of the hormone cream could rub off on that person. It is a good idea to give transdermal hormones time to be thoroughly absorbed in order to avoid transferring them to someone else.

One last note about transdermals. There has been a great deal of confusion about products called "wild-yam creams" that reportedly work like hormone creams. Wild yam does contain a substance, diosgenin, that is used in the laboratory to make natural replacement hormones. However, your body cannot convert diosgenin into hormones; this has to be done in a laboratory. Women have been misled into believing that wild yam itself has hormones in it. It doesn't.

Wild-yam creams are fine as moisturizing skin creams. They certainly aren't harmful, but they aren't hormone creams unless they have actual hormones added to them. One woman told us that she was using a wild-yam cream and that it was alleviating her menopausal symptoms. We tested her to see if her hormone levels had gone up. They had. So we tested the cream she was using to see if it had hormones added to it. It did.

Because they are classified as cosmetics, wild-yam creams are not regulated as stringently or as comprehensively as prescription hormone products (see Who Regulates Over-the-Counter Hormone Supplements? on page 110). In some cases, only very small amounts of hormone have been added to these creams, but in today's competitive market, some companies are adding more and more hormones to their products. Now, instead of 2 percent creams, which contain about 20 milligrams of hormone per gram (about one-quarter teaspoon), we are seeing products with hormone levels as high as 5 percent (50 milligrams per quarter-teaspoon), 6 percent (60 milligrams per quarter-teaspoon), and even 10 percent (100 milligrams per quarter-teaspoon).

There is a wide array of these wild-yam and hormone-containing

WHO REGULATES OVER-THE-COUNTER
HORMONE SUPPLEMENTS?

After a long and arduous battle, the U.S. Congress passed the Dietary Supplement Health and Education Act (DSHEA) in 1994. This groundbreaking law defined *dietary supplements* as "vitamins, minerals, herbs or other botanicals, amino acids, and supplementary dietary substances, and their concentrates, metabolites, constituents, extracts and ingredients," and it officially classified dietary supplements as foods, not drugs. Drugs are subject to the control of the U.S. Food and Drug Administration (FDA), which defines a *drug* as any substance that "alters the structure or function of the human body" or is intended to "treat, prevent, cure, or mitigate disease."

Since the DSHEA was passed, the burden of proof concerning the potential toxicity of substances sold as dietary supplements now rests with the FDA, not the manufacturers who make the products or the retailers who sell them. As a result, the number of products now available over the counter has mushroomed. In order for the Food and Drug Administration to challenge the over-the-counter (OTC) status of any of these supplements, it must prove that the supplement is not safe. This change in the law means more freedom for consumers to pursue health-care alternatives of their own choosing, but it also means less regulation of new products entering the market.

While there are many safe and effective dietary supplement products being offered for sale, not all the products flooding the market have been held to the highest standards before being marketed to consumers. Before you go into a store and reach for the latest, greatest new pill or cream, it is important to know as much as possible not only about the supplement itself but also about the company that manufacturers it. Only in this way can you make the most informed choices about all of the products you are going to put in your body.

As a result of the DSHEA, some of the dietary supplements now more readily available over the counter in the United States are hormone products, including melatonin, DHEA, androstenedione, pregnenolone, and progesterone cream. Many of the companies that manufacture and sell these products are reputable, and their products are of high quality. However, when you are taking hormones, it is important to know how much you are taking. Because of the varying contents of these products and your own individual response to them, it is always important to know what your hormone levels are before you start using them and to monitor your levels to see how you are responding and how your needs might be changing.

creams available now. You can buy ones containing progesterone, estrogen, and DHEA, all available over the counter in health-food stores and through catalogues. They can be very potent medications, yet many women are using them without the assistance or advice of a physician. Because these hormone creams are considered "natural," in some ways like nutritional supplements and vitamins, women believe they are completely safe to use. We have found that some women who use these creams have hormone levels that range from 10 to an alarming 100 times their normal physiologic levels.

Here's something else to consider. The labels on these over-the-counter creams generally recommend doses that are described as one-quarter to one-half teaspoon twice a day. But what does that actually mean? First of all, you have to know what concentration of hormone a cream contains. If you don't, you have no way of knowing how many milligrams of hormone you are getting. Therefore, you have no way of knowing if the recommended dose contains the amount you need. In addition, the cream bases vary widely in weight and other qualities. One-quarter teaspoon of cream should weigh about a gram, but it doesn't always. If you apply a quarter-teaspoon and you are expecting to get a specific amount of medication—for example, 25 milligrams—your dosage could easily be off by as much as 25 percent simply because of the weight of the cream. When you are talking about hormones, or any other medication for that matter, a miscalculation of 25 percent is substantial. In contrast, prescription creams give you precise dosages, so you always know exactly how much of a hormone you are using.

We advocate using hormone products with a doctor's advice and prescription. If you have chosen to use a hormone cream you have purchased over the counter on your own, without the assistance of a physician, at the very least we think you should consider testing your hormone levels to see what is happening.

Even though patches and creams both fall within the transdermal category, they work differently. We think they are both excellent ways for many women to take advantage of HRT. They are convenient and easy to use. It is easy to individualize the dosage with creams. Creams must be applied daily, generally twice a day. A patch application, on the other hand, can last from three to seven days. And most pharmaceutical patches still come only in standard doses. However, years of research and development have finally given us customized natural replacement hormone patches that address the individuality of each woman's needs. As we have seen, the dosage that works for one woman can be too much or too little for another. The adhesives used in patches can cause irritation and allergic reactions in some women. Patch adhesives vary from company to company, however, so if one bothers you, you can try another.

SYMPTOMS AS A HORMONAL BAROMETER

As you can see, the way you take replacement hormones makes a difference. It is not only the dosage but also the delivery system that can influence how HRT affects you. If a hormone dose is too high for you, or a delivery system raises your hormone levels too much, too quickly, you can experience side effects. This doesn't mean you have to give up on HRT, however. It just means you may have to reevaluate your program. Knowing how you are responding to HRT allows you to make decisions based on what works best for you and what is the most comfortable to use. Monitoring your hormone levels and individualizing your hormone replacement allow you to enjoy all the substantial benefits of hormone replacement without side effects.

If you are having physical signs and symptoms of perimenopause or menopause, you have a kind of barometer that tells you yes, your hormone levels may be low. If you begin hormone replacement and your symptoms go away, that is yet another kind of barometer that tells you your program is probably working for you. But how you feel is not necessarily the best way to determine whether you need HRT. Nor is it a reliable way of knowing which replacement hormones you need, or how much of them you should be taking. One of the most important reasons for considering HRT is the protection it can provide from chronic degenerative disease, regardless of how you feel.

As long as you have regular menstrual cycles, your hormones are generally providing you with optimum protection against disease, especially osteoporosis and heart disease. But this is not always the case. Some women can have regular cycles and still have declining hormone levels. When you go through menopause—whether you experience symptoms or not—your hormone levels can also be declining (not every woman's hormones decline at the same rate, or at the same time). Even though many women go through menopause quite easily, without ever experiencing a hot flash, they may still be at risk for osteoporosis and heart disease. Low hormone levels do not always manifest themselves in uncomfortable symptoms. And neither does osteoporosis. This is why homone-level testing is so important.

We have spoken with many women taking conventional HRT who tell us they have never had a bone scan. This means they don't know whether they are at risk for osteoporosis, although they are taking potent medications for it as if they were. It also means that no one is following up to see whether their therapy is having any effect on their bones. Many menopausal and postmenopausal women who are not on hormone replacement have never had a bone scan, either—though the statistics on osteoporosis indicate that maybe they should.

The rate at which your bone is remodeling itself and the effectiveness of your treatment are key factors in the prevention and management of osteoporosis. In the next chapter, we will discuss the options available for determining the health of your bones. We will look at how you can protect your bones by learning what your rate of bone loss is and whether your HRT is effectively slowing it down.

9

Protection for Your Bones

One of the main health concerns women have is osteoporosis, a disease that can rob bones of their strength and leave them more vulnerable to fracture. Osteoporosis gives no warning signals until it is too late and a fracture occurs. A dowager's hump doesn't happen overnight. It is an insidious process in which the vertebrae of the lower back gradually begin compressing together. When they can no longer support the weight of the spine, the interior sides of the vertebrae collapse in on themselves. Nerves are pinched, the abdomen is compressed, and internal organs suffer as the upper back begins to curve. Knowing what is going on with your bones gives you the edge on keeping them healthy and strong.

The only way you can know if you are losing bone mass and need treatment to stop it is to have certain diagnostic tests performed. For many years, the gold standard for testing bone mineral density (BMD) has been dual-energy x-ray absorptiometry (DEXA). More recently, the ultrasonographic bone densitometry test, which uses sound waves to assess BMD, was added to the list of effective tools for measuring the status of your bones. Knowing your bone mineral density is an important factor in determining the current status of your bones and whether you are at risk for osteoporosis (or already have it).

As important and valuable as these tests are in the diagnosis and treatment of osteoporosis, however, BMD tests cannot provide a complete picture of what is happening to your bones. Neither of these methods can be used to determine the rate at which your bones are currently thinning. And we now know that determining your rate of bone loss is a key factor in assessing your osteoporosis risk. It is also important in deciding whether you need treatment and, if so, when it is best to begin it. BMD tests are a way of knowing what has already happened to your bones, not what is actually happening to them right now. In the past, there was no way to measure the actual rate of bone loss. Nor was there a way to determine whether a woman's treatment was actually having an effect on her rate of loss. Fortunately, there now is a test that can give you that information.

IMPORTANT PIECES OF THE PICTURE

Bones are constantly remodeling themselves. In a very active process, old bone cells are destroyed and new bone cells grow to take their place. The remodeling of your bones is a *coupled event*. In other words, the two processes—breaking down and building up—go hand in hand. Bone loss occurs when old bone cells are discarded faster than new cells can be created. If this continues at a high rate over a long period of time, the bone that breaks down doesn't get replaced. Eventually, you end up with bones that are fragile and weak and much more vulnerable to injury.

We now know that the bones that are subjected to the most demand get the most rebuilding. For example, if you don't get enough walking exercise, your hipbones are not going to be triggered to remodel at a normal rate. We also know that bone loss can occur at different rates in different locations in your body. If you don't walk enough but, on the other hand, you do use your arms quite a bit for heavy lifting, your forearms may be fine, while your leg bones and hips may not be getting enough of the exercise they need.

Approximately 10 percent of your bone is remodeled every year. If, over a ten-year period, you add another 2 to 5 percent of bone loss to your normal rate every year—without adding the proper ratio of bone formation—you can see how difficult it will be for your bones to catch up. Another way you can look at it is like this: Over the years, you have been putting money away for your retirement, and you have built up a nest egg. This is your bone mineral density. Now you are ready to retire. Since you no longer have as much money coming in, you have to start withdrawing from your nest egg to live on. This is your bone-remodeling process. If you continue to spend faster than you replenish your funds, then your bank account is going to be depleted. This is bone loss. If, however, you closely monitor your rate of cash flow and keep yourself on a budget, you can protect your resources. This is knowing what your rate of bone loss is so you can take measures to slow it down.

Bone Mineral Density Tests

The dual-energy x-ray absorptiometry, or DEXA, bone-density scan is a noninvasive procedure that exposes you to about the same amount of radiation as a cross-country airplane trip. It measures the density of the bones in your hip, spine, and forearm, and compares this to the bone of a woman at peak bone mass. A woman achieves peak bone mass when she is between the ages of twenty-five and thirty-five. After age thirty-five, she begins losing bone slowly (at a rate of up to 1 percent a year) until she reaches menopause. At menopause, she begins a ten-year cycle during which she loses bone at an accelerated rate (2 to 5 percent a year). At the end of that cycle, bone loss then slows down again to 1 percent a year.

A normal DEXA result would tell you that your bones are "less than one standard deviation" below peak bone mass. What does that mean? If you think of peak bone mass as a measuring cup, and standard deviations as amounts that are missing from the cup, then less than one standard deviation means your cup is full, or nearly full, which is good. A standard deviation of 2.5 yields a diagnosis of osteoporosis. If you are at 2.5 or more, then your measuring cup is less than three-quarters full, which means your bones are greatly at risk of fracture. In fact, studies have shown that if you are at 2.7, your fracture risk increases threefold.

Recently approved by the FDA for testing bone mineral density, the ultrasonographic bone densitometry test is rapidly gaining in popularity among physicians and patients. By measuring the transmission of high-frequency sound waves through your calcaneus (heel) bone, the ultra-sound test is able to quickly give you an assessment of your bones. Unlike the DEXA, this test does not involve x rays. It is painless, nonin-vasive, and fast (it takes about one minute) and is done while you are seated with your foot resting comfortably in the ultrasound device. Test results are available immediately. This makes it possible for your bone mineral density test to be done quickly and easily, right in your health-care practitioner's office.

Whether you have a DEXA or an ultrasonographic bone densitome-try, knowing how much bone you have lost is important in assessing the health of your bones. However, it is not all the information you need. It still tells you only what has already happened to your bones, not what is happening right now. In order to properly manage your resources, you need to know what is going on with your bones right now.

Bone-Resorption Testing: An Investment Counselor for Your Bones

The deoxypyridinoline, or Dpd, test measures your present rate of *bone resorption* (the rate at which bones are being broken down). In much the same way that a saliva test tells you what is going on with your hor-mones, the Dpd test tells you what is happening to your bones, right now. If you are on hormone replacement, a Dpd test can effectively monitor your therapy and tell you how your rate of bone loss is re-sponding to your therapy. If you know what is happening right now, as opposed to what has already happened, you are in a better position to take preventive measures before bone loss accelerates to become osteoporosis.

Here's how it works. The Dpd test measures levels of a substance called deoxypyridinoline, or Dpd, in urine. Dpd is a product of the breakdown of a type of collagen found in your bones. As a result of the bone-breakdown process, Dpd is excreted unmetabolized in urine. Dpd is a very specific marker of bone breakdown, and the Dpd bone-resorption test is very effective in measuring it. Monitoring your rate of bone loss is as important to your bone health as saliva testing, individualizing, and monitoring are to your hormone replacement therapy. Just as saliva test-ing gives you a picture of what is going on with your hormones, a bone-resorption test tells you what is going on with your bones. It can clearly show you whether you are a candidate for HRT.

If your rate of bone loss is high, then your risk for osteoporosis and bone fracture is high. If you decide to begin hormone replacement therapy, follow-up Dpd tests can tell you whether your HRT is effectively slowing your rate of bone loss. A Dpd score of less than 6.5 nM/mM is considered normal, based on test results for healthy men and pre-menopausal nonpregnant women. A score above 6.5 indicates rapid bone breakdown and increased fracture risk.

When your doctor prescribes a Dpd bone-resorption test for you, you can take the test at home, just as you would with a saliva hormone test. Bones remodel at a higher rate while you are sleeping than they do during the day when you are active. So to get the most accurate picture of what is going on with your bones, the ideal collection time for your urine sample is your first or second urination of the day. The sample goes in its own container and into the mail, just like your saliva sample.

Studies suggest that deoxypyridinoline levels can be used to predict whether you are likely to fracture a bone. By using Dpd with a bone-density test, your doctor can fully assess the status of your bones and the rate at which they are changing. That means you know the whole story about your bones, which enables you to make the most informed decisions about treatment.

DEOXYPYRIDINOLINE AND HRT

Once you and your doctor get your Dpd bone-resorption test results back, you can begin to make decisions about whether you need hormone replacement intervention therapy. If you do choose hormone replacement, you can begin to assess within three months how the therapy is working. Further monitoring can then be done at six- or twelve-month intervals, and your therapy can be adjusted whenever necessary based on an accurate assessment of your response. You never have to question whether you are taking enough of a hormone to protect your bones. Nor do you have to wonder whether your hormones are protecting your bones. You will know exactly what is happening. Let's look at how saliva testing, the Dpd test, and hormone replacement therapy work together in practice.

Valerie's Story

Sometimes a Dpd test result can come as a surprise. Valerie is 67 and feeling as fit as a fiddle. She had no real discomforts with her menopause. She was certain that her hormone levels were fine and that her bones were strong and healthy. During her routine physical, Valerie agreed to have both a saliva hormone and a Dpd test—more out of curiosity than concern. Valerie's test results gave her some startling information. Her hormone levels were low, and at 10.4 nM/mM, her Dpd result was very high.

Valerie's test results suggested that she could use estrogen replacement to help slow down her bone-remodeling process. She decided to try it. After three months on 0.25 milligrams of estradiol and 50 milligrams of progesterone, both taken twice a day, Valerie's estradiol and progesterone levels went up to right within her target range. And Valerie was particularly pleased to learn that her Dpd result had gone down to 7.4 nM/mM. Six months later, it was even better, down to 5.2 nM/mM. This showed the effectiveness of her therapy and a substantial decrease in her rate of bone metabolism.

Brenda's Story

Not every woman breezes through her menopause as Valerie seemed to. Take Brenda, who is 55 years old. Her menopausal symptoms were very challenging. She had intractable hot flashes and night sweats, unrelenting insomnia, and bouts of depression that rendered her completely inactive. Brenda also suffered from stress urinary incontinence—every time she sneezed or coughed, she leaked a little urine. That was both irritating and embarrassing for her.

Before Brenda began her menopause at age 51, she was a very social, happy woman. She considered herself fit—she went to the gym three times a week—and she and her husband liked getting away on little excursions at least once a month. Her menopausal discomforts changed a lot of that. At first, she tried conventional hormone replacement, but it was unsuccessful. Her symptoms worsened, and she had an overall feeling that something wasn't quite right. Her doctor at the time tried several standard HRT protocols, but none of them worked. He really didn't know what else to do. That was over three years ago.

Brenda's new doctor is well versed in individualizing and customizing hormone replacement. He also regularly uses Dpd testing to assess a woman's bone health. Even though Brenda was reluctant to try HRT again, her test results and her doctor's confidence in this new individualized approach to hormone restoration encouraged Brenda to give it a try. Brenda started with 0.5 milligrams of estradiol twice daily, plus 100 milligrams of oral progesterone in the morning and another 200 milligrams at night for twelve days out of each month. Brenda's doctor warned her that this might bring her menstrual cycles back. Brenda said she didn't mind; she thought that would be preferable to all the other symptoms she was suffering from. Her doctor also suggested that Brenda go back to exercising in the gym and to walking twenty to thirty minutes at least three times a week. Because Brenda's DHEA and testosterone levels were both low, he also started Brenda on 10 milligrams of DHEA twice a day.

Within the first month of beginning her program Brenda felt like a new woman. The only symptom that didn't seem to go away was her stress urinary incontinence. Her doctor added a 0.5-milligram estriol suppository to be used twice a week, on Saturday and Wednesday. Almost immediately, her incontinence was gone. Brenda was able to resume her life and she was very happy. All of her hormone levels went up to within the normal range. Both her Dpd score and her cortisol level went down, which demonstrated that Brenda's rate of bone metabolism may have been high because of the stress she was experiencing over her menopausal symptoms. After six months on her new individualized therapy, Brenda's Dpd result went down to 6.8 nM/mM, and by the end of the year it was 4.6 nM/mM.

Roxanne's Story

Bone loss does not affect only menopausal and postmenopausal women. Any woman can have bone loss; there are other factors that can trigger it. A woman with an eating disorder like bulimia or anorexia nervosa, for example, can have a high bone-metabolism rate as her body struggles to find the nutrients it needs. Young athletes, who put continuous stress on their bones and their hormones in an attempt to overdevelop themselves while they are still growing, also are at risk for increased bone loss.

Roxanne is only 20 years old. She is a highly competitive marathon runner. Recently, Roxanne suffered a stress fracture in one of her shins.

When she had her hormone levels and her rate of bone resorption tested, the results were startling. Roxanne's bones were breaking down very rapidly.

Because of her unusually low hormone levels, Roxanne's doctor questioned her about her menstrual cycle. Roxanne admitted that since she had started running, at the age of fifteen, she had had periods only very sporadically. When she did have a cycle, she had terrible PMS symptoms—anxiety, crying for no reason, food cravings, abdominal bloating, and breast tenderness. Because Roxanne is so young, her doctor consulted with a pharmacist trained in individualizing hormone prescriptions. Together they decided on a regimen that would help her cycle regularly. She would take estradiol once a day, every day, plus progesterone on days fourteen through twenty-eight. Within the first two months, Roxanne began having a regular period, but without all of her PMS symptoms. In three months, her Dpd was down to 7.9 nM/mM. In six months, it was down to 5.6 nM/mM, and Roxanne was happily back to the track.

FOR OLDER WOMEN, participating in a regular exercise program is a good thing. There are many studies now suggesting that regular exercise has a positive effect on your bones. But excessive exercise can accelerate your rate of bone loss. As we saw in Chapter 2, strenuous exercise can raise cortisol levels. This in turn accelerates the bone-breakdown process. High cortisol levels also can prevent ovulation. If you aren't ovulating, you may not be menstruating, and if you are not having menstrual cycles, you may not be producing enough estrogen, which can also upset the whole process of bone remodeling. Our studies have shown us that women with high cortisol levels also tend to have high Dpd results.

COMPREHENSIVE BONE CARE

Bone remodeling is a tightly coupled process, which means that each phase of the process affects the other. If one phase is out of synch, then the whole process will be out of synch. Doing a bone-resorption test is the best way to begin a comprehensive bone-care program. If you combine bone-resorption testing with a BMD evaluation, you will have an even more complete picture of the status of your bones. It is important to remember that once bone loss has been detected, it can be slowed and even stopped.

Once you know what is happening with your bones, you can make decisions about what action to take. Hormone replacement therapy may be the most natural solution. Hormones stimulate your bone-remodeling process naturally, ensuring that the proper ratio is maintained between building up and breaking down.

While hormone replacement therapy may be the most effective way to prevent and treat osteoporosis, it is not the only way. There are new drugs on the market called *bisphosphonates* that are designed to help treat osteoporosis. One example is alendronate (Fosamax). These drugs work by incorporating synthetic bone into the lattice structure of your bone. This does help to protect your bone from the osteoclasts, the cells that break down bone. How effective bisphosphonates will be at preventing osteoporosis in the long term is not yet known. But when you use bisphosphonates, you are not affecting the entire remodeling process. In some ways, it is like trying to fix a cavity in a tooth without first getting rid of the decay. You are, in effect, protecting the bone from what is breaking it down, but you aren't doing anything to build it back up. If you don't replace the bone that has been broken down with new bone cells, your bones are not going to be as strong as they should be. And although biphosphonates may be helpful in reducing bone turnover, they only address bone issues. They do not offer the multiple benefits of HRT.

There is extensive evidence that HRT can protect your health. Of the 50 million women who will be in menopause in the coming decade, only a small percentage even know about individualized, customized hormone replacement therapy using natural hormones and bone-resorption testing. We want to change that. We want all women to know what all of their options are for the safest, most comprehensive hormone care there is.

When it comes to effective hormone replacement therapy, the key is individuality and variability. We have looked at the individuality of hormonal profiles, hormonal needs, and the ability to absorb, process, and utilize hormone supplementation. We have explored the variables involved in testing procedures, products, and hormone replacement protocols. In the next chapter, we are going to take a closer look at the most changeable variable of them all: you.

10

YOUR LIFESTYLE AND
YOUR HORMONES

We have seen how changeable hormones can be. One hormone can become another, and hormone levels can change at different times of the day, at different times of the month, and at different times of your life. During your life, you change, too. In fact, everything about you changes. Your diet, your stress level, your exercise routine, even your physical condition can all change from one day to the next, from one year to the next. Each of these changes can have an impact on your hormones.

Let's take a moment to consider the kind of person you are. Maybe you are a person who likes to be busy all the time, or maybe you're someone who likes living life at a more leisurely pace. Are you a person who worries, or one who takes each moment as it comes? How about discipline—are you the kind of person who makes resolutions and sticks to them, or do you think resolutions are for the birds? What about your diet—are you conscious of what you eat, or do you like to eat whatever sounds good at the moment? How do you feel about change—do you welcome it or resist it?

You are probably wondering what all these questions have to do with your hormones. They have a great deal to do with them, because their answers can reveal a lot about you and your lifestyle. There is more than enough scientific evidence now to suggest that one of the most important keys to longevity is a healthy lifestyle. Stress reduction, exercise, and a healthy low-fat, high-fiber diet can have a positive effect on you, your hormones, and your hormonal balance.

When you think about whether or not your lifestyle is a healthy one, some of the first questions you might ask yourself are:

- *Am I stressed out?* If the answer is yes, does that necessarily mean that the stress in your life is bad for you? Is there good stress and bad stress? And how much stress is too much?
- *Am I getting enough exercise?* Do you know exactly what the right amount of exercise is, or the right kind? Or even if there *is* a right kind?
- *Am I eating right?* What about your eating habits? Do you know exactly what a well-balanced diet is? Did you answer yes to this question because you eat lots of wholesome, healthy foods? And if you do, does that mean you are guaranteed health, longevity, and hormonal happiness? What about coffee or alcohol—if you consume these things, should you give them up? There's a lot to consider.
- *Am I getting enough sleep?* Women need eight to nine hours of sleep per day for optimum health, yet most get by on less than six and a half hours of sleep during the week and seven hours on weekends. Job stress, family stress, and that "not enough hours in the day" feeling can all contribute to a woman's sleepless nights. Chronic sleeplessness increases cortisol levels. Increased cortisol can cause insomnia. What's a woman to do?

Of all the types of research studies there are, the ones we refer to as lifestyle studies are the hardest to do. The effects of stress, exercise, diet, antioxidants, and vitamins just cannot be scrutinized to the degree that hormone-replacement studies can. In fact, there really haven't been any long-term studies of people who have made controlled, significant changes in their lifestyle and then monitored their hormonal profiles. Think of all the variables that would be involved in that kind of study: Everyone in it would have to eat exactly the same food, do exactly the same kind of exercise for the same amount of time, and use the same stress-reduction techniques for the same kind of stress. Add to that such factors as gender, age, size, and temperament, and you can see why lifestyle studies are so challenging to do.

WHAT'S STRESS GOT TO DO WITH IT?

Diet, exercise, stress, and all the other things that fall into the general category of "lifestyle" do affect your hormonal profile. Lifestyle is one of many reasons why individualizing and monitoring your hormone replacement program is so important.

Table 10.1 illustrates the hormone levels and Dpd bone-resorption test scores of four women whose lives involve high levels of stress. These four women are all about the same age, and they all have busy, intense lives. They are all high-energy women who thrive on being "on the go." There are also some striking differences among them.

Enid: Active and Health-Conscious

Enid was 49 years old. She was five feet tall and weighed a little under 100 pounds. Other than an occasional hot flash, Enid felt terrific most of the time. She prided herself on her healthy lifestyle: She got up and jogged a few miles every morning, ate yogurt and granola for breakfast, worked a nine-to-five job, took breaks, ate a low-fat tofu burger for lunch, had an "organic" dinner at seven o'clock, watched the ten o'clock news, meditated, and was in bed by eleven. Oh, and she took at least two vacations every year with her husband of thirty years.

It seemed as if Enid might have the answer to well-balanced hormones, healthy aging, and longevity. Yet her saliva hormone test results showed that, in fact, all of her sex steroid hormone levels were below the range that provides the most protection. Worse, Enid's Dpd test suggested she was beginning to metabolize bone fairly rapidly. Both Enid's mother and grandmother had had wrist fractures when they were in their late sixties. Even though Enid was enjoying her life, had only a few menopausal hot flashes to contend with, and seemed to be doing everything "right," her test results, body type, and family history indicated she could be at risk for osteoporosis.

Based on her test results, it seemed that hormone replacement would be appropriate for Enid. She managed her stress quite well, and her hor-

	Estradiol	Progesterone	Testosterone	DHEA	Cortisol	Dpd
TABLE 10.1 HORMONE AND DEOXYPYRIDINOLINE (DPD) LEVELS OF FOUR WOMEN WITH HIGH STRESS LEVELS						
Enid	0.6 pg/ml	0.07 ng/ml	22 pg/ml	39 pg/ml	4.8 ng/ml	8.5 nM/mM
Mary	3.1 pg/ml	0.2 ng/ml	32 pg/ml	143 pg/ml	11.4 ng/ml	9.6 nM/mM
Louisa	0.5 pg/ml	0.05 ng/ml	18 pg/ml	32 pg/ml	4.9 ng/ml	5.8 nM/mM
Pamela	0.5 pg/ml	0.02 ng/ml	14 pg/ml	24 pg/ml	0.1 ng/ml	9.3 nM/mM

mone levels were okay, but her family history of bone fracture suggested she might want to protect herself by keeping her hormone levels a little higher.

Enid made no substantial changes in her life other than beginning an individualized hormone replacement program. Her doctor prescribed a 0.35-milligram estradiol tablet and one-eighth teaspoon of 2 percent progesterone cream (supplying 10 milligrams per dose), both to be used twice a day. After a month, Enid had her levels retested to see if this dosage was appropriate for her. It was. Her estradiol level was at 1.8 pg/ml and her progesterone was at 0.3 ng/ml, both right within the range that should provide Enid with bone protection. After six months, her condition was the same, but by the end of a year she had completely stopped cycling and her hormone levels had dropped a bit, even though she was on hormone replacement. Her doctor suggested a slight increase in her dosage, to 0.5 milligrams of estradiol and one-eighth teaspoon of 3 percent progesterone cream twice a day, and when she was tested again, both her estradiol and progesterone levels were just right.

Mary: Busy Single Mother

Mary was 49 years old. She was five feet, four inches tall and weighed approximately 120 pounds. Like Enid, Mary was busy all the time. She was a single working mother with three children, and she was attending night school to get a degree in computer programming. Mary did aerobics four or five times a week, was a Cub Scout den mother, and also managed to do volunteer work at the local retirement home. Her diet was fairly typical— mostly home-cooked meals with only the occasional pizza or burger and fries when she was on the run.

When Mary told her doctor she was interested in hormone replacement therapy, it was because she was experiencing some forgetfulness and insomnia. Her menstrual cycles had been tapering off for nearly a year, but she was still having light periods almost every other month. Mary's saliva hormone levels told a very different story from Enid's. Most of Mary's hormone levels looked very good, well within the range you would expect to see in a woman who is still menstruating. However, her cortisol level was very, very high and so was her Dpd. These levels indicated that stress was having a physiologic effect on her.

What was going on with Mary? Was it her busy life that was causing her forgetfulness? Or her stress that was keeping her up at night? Mary claimed that she was very happy with her life, that she enjoyed everything she was doing. But we can see that Mary's stress was affecting her cortisol level dramatically, though her other hormone levels seemed to be fine.

Because Mary's hormone levels were still fairly high, hormone replacement was not appropriate for her. She was going to have to do something about her cortisol level, though, and her Dpd. That meant taking measures to reduce stress and protect her bones. Mary decided that she would begin a yoga class in place of her aerobics and that she would stay for the meditation that was offered after the class. She cut back on the number of units she was taking in school and started using her extra time for some stressless activities like walking in the park, reading for pleasure instead of just for school, and listening to music. Mary invited another Cub Scout mother to help out with the group. She also made a conscious effort to include more calcium-rich foods in her diet and started taking 1,500 milligrams of supplemental calcium each day.

At the end of six months, Mary's cortisol level was 7.7 ng/ml and her Dpd was 7.4 nM/mM, both noticeably lower. At the end of a year, her cortisol was 4.5 ng/ml and her Dpd 5.9 nM/mM, both well within the normal range. She was now, however, beginning to experience hot flashes and mild headaches. Her saliva test showed that, with the waning of her menstrual cycles, her progesterone and estradiol levels were now declining slightly. Mary didn't want to take hormone replacement yet. She decided to recheck her levels again in a few months and to watch her symptoms to see how they progressed.

Louisa: High-Stress and Loving It

Louisa was 47 years old and the chief executive officer of a large financial-planning corporation. She was five feet, seven inches tall, weighed 160 pounds, and was still menstruating. Louisa started her morning with a large mug of coffee. On her way to work, she would eat a quickie energy bar in the car while talking on her cell phone. She usually popped a soda about brunch time, skipped lunch, and ate take-out food for dinner. Louisa worked fourteen hours a day most days, had no time for exercise, and absolutely no time for meditation or relaxation. On the weekends, she usually tried to catch up on her sleep and take in some form of social activity.

Louisa loved her job and the financial security it had given her, but she had started to experience cold chills, clammy hands, and panic attacks. She also had fibrocystic breasts and uterine fibroids, and her libido seemed to have disappeared. During her routine physical checkup, Louisa complained to her doctor that she didn't feel like her old self—that she was having to push herself more to keep up her usual fast pace. Could it be that Louisa's lifestyle was having a negative impact on her hormone levels? Possibly. But she loved her job. She even loved her stress. Doesn't that count for something?

Apparently it does. Her cortisol level was low, which was very good and indicated that for the most part Louisa was not "stressed out." And her Dpd showed a normal rate of bone metabolism. However, all of Louisa's sex steroid hormone levels would have been low even for a woman much older than Louisa. Were Louisa's symptoms just the tip of an iceberg? Would there be more to come if she didn't slow down? Should Louisa make dramatic changes in her life—change her diet, get more exercise, maybe even give up her job?

Even though Louisa appeared to be coping with her stress, her hormone levels had declined very rapidly. Louisa was very disheartened that her hormone levels were so low. She told her doctor that she liked her life and didn't want to have to make any changes. Louisa's doctor suggested a comprehensive hormone replacement program to restore her hormone levels, including a 0.05-milligram estradiol patch to be worn every day and replaced weekly. He also prescribed a one-eighth teaspoon of 2 percent progesterone cream to be applied twice a day and 20 milligrams of DHEA and 5 milligrams of testosterone in tablet form to be used once a day.

While he was writing her prescriptions, Louisa's doctor explained to her that too much stress eventually kills the machine and that, over time, her stress would take a toll on her health. He reassured her that when she started her hormone replacement, she would start feeling more like her old self. But he thought he would be remiss not to at least suggest that a reduction in her stress would result in an improvement in her overall health. Giving up coffee would help her fibrocystic breasts. Incorporating some regular exercise and, possibly, some relaxation techniques could only benefit her hormone levels.

Louisa agreed to try to do more than just take her HRT. She knew that in the long run it would be best. When she started taking the hormones, she also gave up drinking coffee and cut her workdays down a bit (which took considerable self-discipline). During the first month, Louisa was full of energy and her libido was back in full bloom. She was feeling great—no more panic attacks, cold chills, or clammy hands. When she was retested, her saliva hormone levels were all well within the target range for a woman her age. And her cortisol and Dpd couldn't have been better. However, Louisa's testosterone level was noticeably higher than it should have been for a woman her age and was approaching a level that could begin to cause her some side effects. Her doctor wasn't quite sure what was happening. He called a pharmacist trained in individualized HRT with some questions about Louisa's dosages. The pharmacist explained to him that Louisa's DHEA was probably cascading into testosterone (see page 37), and suggested that she stop taking both of these hormones and then test again in a month.

While Louisa was off of her DHEA and testosterone, however, she complained that her energy was flagging again and so was her libido. And at the end of the month, her tests showed that she did need both of these hormones. At this point, the pharmacist suggested to Louisa's doctor that she begin therapy again, but at a lower dose of 15 milligrams of DHEA and 2.5 milligrams of testosterone. One month later, Louisa's levels had increased just enough. Her DHEA was at 117 pg/ml and her testosterone at 36 pg/ml. Louisa's hormone levels have since remained balanced and she has been symptom-free, though that may change as she gets closer to menopause.

⌒

ENID, MARY, AND LOUISA all led very high-stress lives, but each coped with stress in different ways. That is the beauty of individuality. All of these women found their lifestyles exciting, challenging, and energizing, and they thrived on this. If they were to go through life at a leisurely pace, they would feel as if they were half-asleep. To be idle, have too much downtime, or not enough success would be a source of negative stress for them. This is, of course, not the case with everyone.

Pamela: Exhausted by Stress

Pamela, 52, hadn't had a menstrual cycle for two years. She was five feet, nine inches tall and weighed 165 pounds. At first glance, Pamela's life seemed to be fairly simple. She had worked at the same job for fifteen years. Her children had both graduated from high school—one had gone off to college and the other was still living at home.

During a routine physical exam, Pam told her doctor she was getting divorced. She was actually looking forward to her freedom, but she was so tired all the time she couldn't seem to enjoy herself. Pam also confided that, even though she was exhausted, she felt anxious, too. And her heart had started fluttering recently. She felt cold most of the time, and her hair seemed to be falling out more than usual. Pam thought she might need hormone replacement.

When Pamela's doctor took her blood pressure, it was 90/50, which is low. This was a little red flag to Pamela's doctor, because her blood pressure had never been that low before. When he went over her chart, he saw that Pam had had several bouts of bronchitis over the last year and had had an unusually hard time fighting them off. He also noted that she had not been menstruating for two years. Pam's doctor ordered a saliva hormone test for her, and, indeed, Pam had very low hormone levels, particularly low DHEA and cortisol, and her Dpd was very high.

In much the same way that high cortisol levels can be an indication that a person is under intense, chronic stress, low morning levels of cortisol can, too. That is because this kind of stress can deplete the adrenal glands. Pamela's low DHEA levels were an indication that her adrenal glands might not be coping with the stress she was under. This let her doctor know that more was going on with Pam than first met his eye. Her test results also showed Pam that, even though she believed she was managing her stress fairly well, it was taking a toll on her.

Pamela and her doctor talked further about what had been going on in her life. She told him that she was relieved to be finally ending her marriage, which had been a terrible hardship on her for many years. Classically, she and her husband had stayed together for the sake of the children, but it was a very unhappy situation for her. Pamela had also been very anxious about her financial future. The company she worked for had merged with a large corporation, and her job had been in jeopardy for months. Her son had been in trouble at college, and, even though she knew it was probably just a reaction to the divorce, it was difficult for her to deal with. On top of that, Pamela's father had died recently after a lengthy illness.

After going over her saliva test results and talking with her further, Pamela's doctor believed she was a good candidate for hormone replacement therapy, though he was concerned that it might not be enough to restore her health. He thought Pamela also needed to make some changes in her life. So her doctor suggested that Pamela make an effort to include more fresh vegetables and fruits in her diet and that she take a daily vitamin and mineral supplement. He further advised her to begin a program of regular but not too strenuous exercise, such as swimming or walking. He also suggested she incorporate more pleasurable experiences into her life, to calm her and to bring the enjoyment back into her life.

But Pamela wasn't sure she wanted to take hormones. First, she wanted to try all the lifestyle changes her doctor suggested. For the first month, she was religious about her diet, exercise, and relaxation. She started feeling a little better, but she was still so fatigued she barely had the energy to keep herself on track. When she tested her hormone levels again, there were no noticeable changes. Pamela then conceded and accepted a prescription for 1 milligram of estradiol, 250 milligrams of progesterone, and 3.5 milligrams of testosterone daily. Within days, she began to feel like a new person. She had the energy she needed for her new lifestyle.

At six months, Pamela's hormone levels continued to be in the range most desirable for her, and she was feeling stronger every day. She even started enjoying all the changes she had made in her life. She was very glad her saliva tests had alerted her to the fact that she needed to make them. Her hormone restoration program was revitalizing her health and her life.

As you can see, even though they are all in the same age group and are all leading active, busy lives, each of these women discussed in this section is completely individual in her hormonal profile. That is why an individualized approach to hormone replacement is so important. Only by knowing what is going on, right now, with your hormones and by monitoring your hormonal changes, can you and your doctor learn what the effects of stress on your hormones really are.

THE EFFECTS OF EXERCISE

We all want to feel good about ourselves. And most of us want to live long, healthy, productive lives, but what that means to each of us can be very different. Some women are willing to make lifestyle changes that require discipline and sacrifice; some are not. Some women just want to feel better and be better as quickly and easily as possible. Others love the challenge of working at it. Is one person's way better than another? We don't have the answer to that yet.

We know that exercise can reduce your risk of heart disease, increase your bone density, decrease stress, and make you look and feel better. Research is showing us that exercise can have a positive impact on your hormones. Both male and female high-performance athletes, for example, can experience increases in their testosterone levels. Weight-bearing exercise has also been shown to increase testosterone levels. As with everything else in life, however, how you respond hormonally to exercise depends on your individual physiologic makeup. And not everyone's hormones do respond, no matter how much they exercise. Once again, individuality is the key.

There are many different kinds of exercise programs—weights, aerobics, jogging, walking, yoga, and swimming, to name a few. The positive effects of each are invaluable. They are all good for you in different ways. We don't have enough conclusive scientific evidence yet to assure you that if you do a specific amount of any of these types of activity every day, you will increase or decrease your hormone levels or your need for replacement hormones. We can't tell you whether one exercise is positively better for your hormones than another. How much you weigh, how old you are, what you eat, what kind of metabolism you have, how much rest you get—all of these affect how you respond to exercise. But we do know that strength, flexibility, endurance, and increased cardiovascular performance all contribute to health and well-being and, ultimately, to how you feel about yourself.

Table 10.2 shows the hormone levels and Dpd bone-resorption test scores of three physically active women. Jolene, 41, is a long-distance runner. Grace prefers weight lifting to other forms of exercise. She is 52 years old and very fit. Rita is a swimmer. She is 45 years old. Each of these women exercises strenuously as a regular part of her life. Yet, as you can see, they have very different hormone levels.

Clearly, even though a continuous exercise program can help you maintain your health and your hormonal balance, exercise does not affect all women in exactly the same way. We simply cannot tell you how much exercise to do, or what kind you should choose. The only way we can tell you how your exercise program is affecting your hormone levels is by testing them. If you begin to exercise regularly and stay with it while you are on a hormone replacement program, you can saliva-test your hormone levels to see how you are doing. Your test results can tell you if your exercise regimen is decreasing your need for hormones or enhancing how you respond to the ones you are taking.

THE IMPACT OF DIET

There is substantial scientific evidence to suggest that your diet can affect your hormone levels. But when it comes to the specific influences your diet can have, there are many, many variables to consider. For example, you may have heard that eating soy foods or taking soy supplements can be beneficial to you and to your hormone levels. The most recent scientific information does suggest that soy is probably beneficial, but we are not able to say unequivocally at this point that this is true. The reason soy is heralded as being beneficial to your hormones is that it contains isoflavones. Isoflavones are phytoestrogens, or plant estrogens, that are very similar in chemical structure to human estrogens and are thought to have estrogenic activity in the body. But soy has many isoflavones, not

TABLE 10.2   HORMONE AND DEOXYPYRIDINOLINE (DPD) LEVELS OF THREE PHYSICALLY ACTIVE WOMEN

	Estradiol	Progesterone	Testosterone	DHEA	Cortisol	Dpd
Jolene	0.6 pg/ml	0.06 ng/ml	38 pg/ml	149 pg/ml	4.9 ng/ml	9.2 nM/mM
Grace	0.9 pg/ml	0.08 ng/ml	31 pg/ml	121 pg/ml	4.4 ng/ml	4.8 nM/mM
Rita	2.8 pg/ml	0.3 ng/ml	23 pg/ml	130 pg/ml	3.8 ng/ml	5.4 nM/mM

just one. Before we can say we completely understand all of them and can make definitive statements about how each of them affects our hormones, much more research and testing need to be done.

Many claims are being made that a diet high in phytoestrogens can affect your hormonal balance. We have been studying phytoestrogens for some time, and at this point in our research we can only partially evaluate their hormonal influence. Some of the research we have done with phytoestrogenic herbs has shown us that they can have estrogenic effects. But what does that mean? Just because something has estrogenic effects, that doesn't necessarily mean it will decrease your hot flashes or night sweats, or alleviate any of your other menopausal symptoms. We know that phytoestrogens can bind with your receptors. What we do not know is what effect that has on the body. Remember, the structure of a hormone is very important when it comes to your receptors.

The phytoestrogen/estrogen question is further complicated by the fact that estrogen is not a single hormone but a family of hormones. We do not yet know how (or even if) phytoestrogens affect the levels of the different estrogens in the body. Scientific data that can tell you exactly what impact a diet high in phytoestrogens will have on your hormone levels simply do not exist yet.

Many women have started taking supplements containing phytoestrogenic plant extracts, not only to help eliminate their menopausal symptoms but also, hopefully, to gain protection from heart disease and osteoporosis. Some women who make this choice do so because they want to live as "naturally" as they can; others because they are afraid of the increased cancer risk that has been associated with HRT. Studies have shown that phytoestrogens are great antioxidants, and antioxidants have been shown to be protective of the body, but no studies have conclusively demonstrated that phytoestrogens are associated with a lower risk of breast cancer than replacement hormones are. Nor have any studies proven that phytoestrogens provide protection from heart disease or osteoporosis.

The issue of dietary impact on hormonal balance is an important one. A diet high in fat can affect your estrogen levels in more ways than one. If you eat a high-fat diet, you are likely to have more body fat, which in turn is likely to increase your estrone levels. A high-fat diet can also increase enterohepatic recirculation of your estrogens, which keeps estrogens circulating in your body instead of being eliminated (see page 105). A high-fiber diet, on the other hand, can actually lower your hormone levels. Dietary fiber can literally soak up hormones in your intestinal tract and pass them out in your stool. This prevents them from being recirculated. Japanese women, who tend to eat a diet high in fiber and moderate in fat, generally have only half the circulating estrogens that Western women do.

It is important to understand that if you are perimenopausal, your estrogen level may be increased, either because you have more body fat or because you are consuming high-fat meals. This is at a time when your body is no longer producing a proportionate amount of progesterone, which means your estrogens are no longer working in concert with their protective partner but are very busy on their own. Remember, estrogen is a stimulating hormone. It makes things happen. Too much estrogen without enough progesterone can mean swollen breasts, PMS, and a whole host of other symptoms. If you are experiencing these symptoms, making sure that your diet is high in fiber and low in fat might be very beneficial because it can aid in reducing your level of circulating estrogens.

Scientific information is constantly evolving. Sometimes the things we believe to be good for us turn out, upon further investigation, to be not good at all. Take the case of margarine. For years, science believed that margarine was better for us than butter. Now, however, studies have shown that hydrogenated oils (an ingredient in most margarines) and the trans-fatty acids they contain are, in fact, harmful to us. Eggs are another example. In the not-so-distant past, eggs were looked upon as little cholesterol demons. Now health experts tell us they may be a near-perfect food that—in moderation—is beneficial. Nuts also are foods that were once considered unhealthy, mainly because of their fat content. However, we now know that nuts are high in omega-3 acids, and these fats are actually good for you. The Iowa Women's Health Study and the

Physicians' Health Study found that eating nuts frequently may actually reduce the risk of cardiovascular disease.

In every area of life, our knowledge base is continually growing and changing. And the more we learn, it seems, the more we need to learn. That is why we stress the importance of having as much scientifically proven data as possible before making absolute claims about hormones or hormone replacement therapy.

Just as a healthy diet can aid your hormonal balance, similarly, relaxation and meditation can positively affect hormone levels. Stress reduction can enhance your hormone replacement program. Whether or not thirty minutes of meditation every day will be enough to help you manage your stress and help to balance your hormone levels depends on you. The beauty of saliva testing and individualized hormone replacement is that, if you make changes in your life, you can see if they are making a difference for you. We cannot tell you what kind of stress is good for you or what kind is bad. Nor can we tell you how much stress is too much for you. But you can monitor how your stress is affecting you and what it is doing to your body.

THE IMPORTANCE OF INDIVIDUALITY

Stress reduction, regular exercise, and healthy eating are all good for you. There is no question they can influence your hormone levels. But no one can assure you yet that any single one of them, or any combination of them, will affect your hormones in a specific way. We simply do not have a complete understanding of all the influences that diet, exercise, and stress have on us, although we do know that they result in real chemical changes in the body. We are gaining a better understanding of their impact all the time, but it is certain to be a never-ending area of investigation.

We believe it is beneficial for any woman who is trying to manage her hormones to be more conscious about her lifestyle choices, but we need more scientific research in these areas before we can start writing prescriptions for lifestyle changes that will change your hormone levels. That is yet another reason why individualizing hormone replacement and monitoring your hormone levels is so important. Because saliva testing tells you what is going on, right now, with your hormones, it can help you measure the effects of your lifestyle on your hormones and determine whether you need to make any lifestyle changes. Once you do, it can help you assess whether the changes you make are having a positive effect. If your test results affirm that the changes you have made in your lifestyle are indeed benefiting you and your hormone levels, you may be encouraged to continue doing what is good for you, instead of lapsing into habits that are not.

If you are interested in trying to influence your hormones with your lifestyle, we encourage you to do that. Even minor changes in how you live can alter your need for replacement hormones, whether increasing or decreasing it. What happens while you are on a hormone replacement program depends on your evolving hormonal profile. Many women who are on (or are considering) HRT wonder how long they can, or should, continue taking it. Just like everything else, this depends on you. We believe that because it provides for ongoing diagnosis and monitoring, and is customized to meet your ever-changing needs, individualized hormone restoration is a program you can choose to use for life. The real question may not be how long you should be on hormone replacement, but how you will address your ever-changing needs while you are. In the chapter that follows, we will meet some of the many women who have benefited from an individualized approach to hormone restoration.

11

PUTTING IT ALL TOGETHER

As we have seen, hormone therapy provides a multitude of benefits for many women for a whole variety of reasons. While the one-size-fits-all method has been the most widely prescribed, it has not worked for many women because it does not take each woman's individuality into account. As a result, many women who could benefit greatly from hormone restoration have become discouraged with it or abandoned it completely because it caused intolerable side effects.

Considering how complex your endocrine system and hormonal balance are, doesn't it make sense to find out exactly what is going on with your hormones and what treatment, if any, is right for you, and then to monitor your ever-changing needs? Fortunately, with an individualized approach to HRT, it is possible to fine-tune your hormone replacement program to meet your precise needs. In this chapter, we will look at individualized hormone replacement therapy in action, using the stories of real women who have tried it. As you will see from the experiences of women who have been using saliva testing, individually customized prescription therapy, and hormone-level monitoring, this new approach to HRT is an enormous advance in women's health care.

LANA'S STORY

We have met Lana twice before, in Chapter 3 and Chapter 7. She is the 51-year-old marketing director who was considering pursuing her life-long dream of opening a small nursery but was being held back by a host of menopausal symptoms, including fatigue, mood swings, forgetfulness, insomnia, and a seeming inability to concentrate. She also complained of having lost all interest in sex. When her doctor tested her saliva hormone levels, he suggested that Lana also have a Dpd test.

In fact, it did appear that Lana's hormone levels were low, but that is not all her tests revealed. Lana's Dpd test score was 8.5 nM/mM, which demonstrated that she was metabolizing bone rapidly. Her doctor decided to do an ultrasonographic bone densitometry test right then, and her score on that test was normal: Her bones looked just fine. Lana was confused by these very different bone-test results. Her doctor explained that for a woman her age they were not uncommon. In fact, this was good news; it meant that Lana's bones were in great shape now (giving her a good head start on maintaining their strength), but because she was entering menopause and her hormone levels were declining, her bone-metabolism rate was on the increase. Having these two test results gave Lana the information she needed to decide to intervene in that process and begin hormone replacement in time to preserve the health of her bones.

Lana's doctor prescribed a combination of HRT for her that included 1.5 milligrams of estradiol, 200 milligrams of oral micronized progesterone, and 3 milligrams of testosterone daily. He also recommended that she take a calcium citrate supplement every day and begin a regular exercise program.

At the end of one month, when Lana retested her hormone levels, they were all within the range considered optimal for her health. She was again feeling like her energetic, clear-headed, enthusiastic, and sexy self. At the end of six months, her Dpd score was down to 6.2 nM/mM, which showed that she was no longer metabolizing bone at an accelerated rate. And, yes, Lana did leave her marketing job and buy that small nursery she had always wanted, and she is doing quite well.

JANE ANN'S STORY

Jane Ann, a 49-year old financial planner, relied on a self-care program that included a healthful diet, a regular workout regimen, and a vitamin and mineral supplement to manage her occasional hot flashes. Gradually, however, in spite of everything she was doing on her own, Jane's hot flashes became an all-too-common occurrence. A person who prided herself on keeping details within her grasp, Jane was also noticing a few gaps in memory that concerned her. For example, she would reach a client on the phone and, right after saying hello, forget why she called. Or she would pluck a report from her shelf, search through it, and suddenly be unable to recall what she was looking for.

Due for her routine annual physical exam, Jane Ann decided to discuss her concerns with her doctor. During their conversation, she told him that, along with her other symptoms, she was also feeling close to tears more frequently, often without a reason she could identify, and that she had not had a period for quite a few months. Jane Ann's doctor listened intently and then explained to her that her symptoms, combined with her age and the fact that her cycles seemed to be waning, led him to believe that she was entering menopause and that her estrogen level was low. He gave her a prescription for conventional doses of Premarin and Provera. Within just two weeks Jane Ann was back in her doctor's office, reporting that she felt terrible. Her normally cheerful outlook on life was now bleak; her breasts were very tender; and she felt bloated all the time. She did not understand why her symptoms were now worse.

Having just returned from a seminar on saliva hormone testing and individualized hormone replacement, Jane Ann's doctor decided to take a different course with her. He suggested running a saliva hormone test to measure her free-hormone levels and a Dpd test to see how her bones were doing. After reviewing the results of the saliva measurement, he could see that her estradiol level was indeed above the expected range. The target level for a woman who is still having menstrual cycles is between 3 and 8 pg/ml. At 18.7 pg/ml, Jane Ann's estradiol level was way too high. Her doctor correctly surmised that this was making her symptoms worse. For Jane Ann, the standard dose of Premarin was obviously much too strong.

In order to find the right approach for Jane Ann, her doctor consulted with a pharmacist trained in interpreting saliva hormone test results and individualizing hormone therapy dosages. He then switched her from

Premarin and Provera to natural replacement estradiol and oral micronized progesterone. He explained to Jane Ann that these hormones were identical to those her body produced and assured her that many women have found natural replacement hormones much easier to tolerate than the animal-derived and synthetic varieties. He adjusted her dosages to 0.5 milligrams of estradiol and 100 milligrams of progesterone, to be taken twice a day.

Within a day or two, Jane Ann felt like herself again. A follow-up saliva test thirty days later showed that, indeed, her estradiol level was 3.2 pg/ml and her progesterone level was 0.4 ng/ml, both well within the ranges you would see in a woman who is still menstruating. Jane Ann's hot flashes were under control, she wasn't teary any longer, and she felt like she had her wits about her again.

Jane Ann's first experience with HRT—having standardized dosages of synthetic hormones prescribed without testing of her free-hormone levels—is not unusual. In fact, many women have had this experience, because most physicians still rely on their observation of a woman's symptoms to determine whether she needs hormone therapy or not. Unfortunately, conventional HRT protocols prescribed that way are often unsuccessful. Replacement hormones can cause severe and uncomfortable side effects if they raise a woman's hormone levels too much. And women who have negative reactions to hormone replacement often stop taking it altogether. This is unfortunate. Most of the time, all that is needed is for their doctors to adjust the prescriptions to something more suitable to them. Often, that can mean something as simple as lowering the dosage or changing the delivery system. It is important to note that not all women develop symptoms when their dosages are too high. It is important to monitor exactly what your hormone replacement therapy is doing in your body, because there is no reason to take more of a hormone (or any other medication, for that matter) than you need.

CELESTE'S STORY

When Celeste, a healthy, active 47-year-old, started having her first peri-menopausal symptoms, she decided she was going to try to help herself through "the change." She read books on natural approaches to menopause, adjusted her diet, began an exercise regimen, and took nutritional supple-

ments and herbs. Three months later, she still found herself crying at the drop of a hat; craving foods like pasta, chocolate, and potatoes; and having hotter and hotter hot flashes. One night, her husband sat bolt upright in bed and said, "What's going on with you and the covers? One minute they're on, the next minute they're flying off!"

Celeste continued her search for answers to her premenopausal woes. She found an over-the-counter natural progesterone cream on the Internet. It sounded appealing to her, so she ordered it. When Celeste received her cream she read the instructions and decided that because she was still having periods, even though they were irregular, she should take the dose recommended for a premenopausal woman who is still menstruating. For several weeks, Celeste used the cream this way, with good results: Her mood improved, her food cravings diminished, and she had less frequent hot flashes and more restful sleep. But within a short time, some of her symptoms seemed to be coming back.

This made Celeste wonder if she might be further along in the change than she had originally thought. "Maybe I'm not using enough of the cream," she thought. She decided to try applying more. Almost immediately, Celeste began feeling sleepy all the time, and, on top of everything else, her sex drive was kaput. She was becoming increasingly worried. What if it wasn't the change at all—what if something was really wrong with her? She stopped using the cream and made an appointment with her doctor.

Celeste told her doctor what was happening, and he ordered a blood test of her hormone levels. The results showed that her estrogen and progesterone levels were what you would expect in a woman who is still menstruating. "Your hormones look fine," her doctor told her. "Maybe you're just having a hard time adjusting to the idea that you're approaching 'the change.'" Celeste was puzzled and frustrated. She did not think she was depressed; she intuitively knew something was going on with her hormones.

So Celeste spent a few more late nights on the Internet, where she found some information on saliva hormone testing. She was intrigued enough to call her doctor and ask if saliva testing would be appropriate for her. Although he wasn't familiar with saliva hormone testing and hadn't used it with his other patients, he agreed to review the information Celeste had found. He called her back a few days later and said he was willing to order the saliva hormone test and consider the results. Celeste's saliva hormone test revealed that her progesterone level was 0.03 ng/ml, well below the target range for a woman her age who is still menstruating.

After consulting with a pharmacist who specialized in the interpretation of saliva testing and formulating individualized hormone doses, Celeste's doctor told her that over-the-counter creams can vary widely in the amount of hormone they contain, if they contain any at all. He recommended that a prescription cream be formulated especially for her, so that they both would know exactly how much hormone she was getting. He told Celeste how important it is to monitor the dosage closely. She had not been able to do that effectively when she applied the over-the-counter cream in varying amounts. Celeste began using her prescription cream, and she began feeling better right away.

After a month of using her new, individualized progesterone cream, even though Celeste was feeling quite well, her follow-up saliva test showed that her progesterone level was in fact slightly above the optimum range. This information indicated that her dosage needed to be decreased slightly. Her doctor lowered her dosage again, this time recommending that she use only 20 milligrams of progesterone cream a day, divided into two one-eighth-teaspoon doses containing 10 milligrams each. Celeste felt terrific using this amount, and thirty days later her follow-up saliva test showed that her progesterone level was 0.4 ng/ml—right within her target range.

Three very important things were accomplished in Celeste's case. First, she and her doctor were able to obtain a precise picture of her free-hormone levels using saliva testing. Second, together with a pharmacist trained in this specialized approach to hormone replacement therapy, Celeste's doctor was able to adjust her dosage to precisely what she needed, the amount that was just right for her body. Third, Celeste and her doctor have an ongoing means of monitoring her progress with follow-up testing, and they can adjust her dosage as needed. As Celeste's body continues to change, her hormonal requirements may change, too. If they do, she and her doctor can respond with more information and less guesswork.

ELLY'S STORY

Elly, a 65-year-old woman whose 89-year-old mother had become increasingly frail and dependent, had been her mother's primary caregiver for the last eight years. At first, it was not that difficult for Elly to take care of her mother. They had always been very close, and Elly loved her very much. She couldn't bear the thought of having to institutionalize her. However, "Mum's" condition was progressive, and over the years Elly's mother became more and more difficult for Elly to cope with, both physically and emotionally.

When Elly's case was reviewed by her nurse practitioner, Elly was experiencing extreme fatigue, night sweats, heart palpitations, depression, and insomnia. Since she found it difficult to find anyone to come in and help care for her mother, Elly was pleased to be able to take her saliva hormone and Dpd tests at home, early in the morning, while her mother was sleeping.

As might have been expected, most of Elly's hormone levels were at the low end of the desired range for a postmenopausal woman. This was not unusual, considering her age and the fact that she was not then using hormone replacement—and the significant stress she was under. But at 11.9 ng/ml, Elly's cortisol level was alarmingly high, and at over 8.5 nM/mM, so was her Dpd.

Remember, cortisol is your stress hormone, and a high cortisol level is often associated with increased bone breakdown. The normal level for cortisol at 8:00 A.M. is below 8 ng/ml. The fact that Elly's was nearly 50 percent above normal indicated that the chronic stress of her role as caregiver for her mother could be taking a physical toll on her. Her nurse practitioner immediately ordered a DEXA bone-density test for Elly so that she could more fully assess the health of Elly's bones. The DEXA result showed that she had already experienced a significant amount of bone loss.

A discussion about hormone replacement was very important for Elly. A pharmacist specializing in individualized hormone replacement therapy was able to suggest a program for her that would be both very easy to use and very effective at alleviating many of her symptoms. Elly would be using a 0.05-milligram estradiol patch. In addition, she would take a 300-milligram timed-release tablet of oral micronized progesterone and a 3.5-milligram testosterone tablet each day.

As Elly found out, the connection between stress and hormones is an important one. And saliva hormone-level testing can often reveal problems that may require other therapies in addition to HRT. With her cortisol level as high as it was, another important line of intervention for Elly was going to be stress management.

Elly's nurse practitioner talked with Elly about her test results and explained how important it would be to consider some form of relaxation and light exercise. In addition to her hormone replacement, Elly took up walking and meditating.

After one month on her new program, Elly was retested. Her hormone levels were now back in the range they were when she was still having her menstrual cycles. Her cortisol was on the way down, which was a good sign; it meant that Elly was managing her stress a little better. She was feeling much stronger and much more able to cope with the rigors of caring for her mother. Unfortunately, she would not be able to regain the bone she had lost before beginning therapy, but after six months on HRT, her Dpd was down to 6.4 nM/mM, a range that suggested Elly was no longer losing bone at such a high rate. This should enable her to better maintain the bone density she does have.

RANDA'S STORY

Randa, a 54-year-old grandmother who regularly baby-sat for her very active 2-year-old twin grandsons, had noticed a real drop in her energy level. Moreover, she seemed to be carrying a few extra pounds she just couldn't shake, no matter how much she exercised. Randa was postmenopausal and had had the good fortune of breezing through her change. She was used to having an abundance of energy, and with the twins around, she really needed it. She felt frustrated and depressed by the fatigue she couldn't explain.

Randa made an appointment with her family doctor and explained to him how tired she was feeling. He talked with her about the demands of chasing two toddlers and asked about her diet and exercise habits. It was, he said, somewhat to be expected that she would feel tired, given that, Monday through Friday, Randa provided loving and attentive care to her grandsons. "I see women twenty years younger than you who are exhausted by their small children," he told her. He suggested she try to incorporate a little more "time out for Grandma" into her daily routine. Randa left his office feeling a little discouraged and still wanting to find a solution to her fatigue.

Then Randa saw an ad in one of her favorite health magazines for the hormone DHEA. It promised new energy and vitality. Thinking it was similar to taking a vitamin or herb, she started taking 25 milligrams of

DHEA each day. She didn't mention it to her doctor. After taking DHEA for about a month, Randa felt great. And yes, she thought she did feel more energetic. However, after three months on DHEA, Randa noticed that even though she had more energy, she now seemed to be more anxious and irritable. She was snapping at the twins more frequently, and she didn't know why—they weren't doing anything different.

This time, Randa made an appointment with her gynecologist. When the gynecologist learned that Randa had been taking DHEA supplements, she ordered a saliva hormone test to take a closer look at Randa's estrogen, progesterone, DHEA, and testosterone levels. The test revealed that Randa's DHEA level was extremely high, at 500 pg/ml, which was probably contributing to why Randa was feeling very energetic. But remember, hormones are interrelated. They can affect one another. Randa's testosterone level also was high—in fact, it was very high. It was 75 pg/ml. Ordinarily, a woman Randa's age would have a saliva testosterone level somewhere in the area of 25 pg/ml. Even a twenty-year-old woman would not normally have a testosterone level exceeding 50 pg/ml. Randa's level was now well above the normal range for any woman.

As we saw in Chapter 3, DHEA is a hormone that cascades into other hormones in the body. In Randa's case, the DHEA she was taking not only raised her DHEA level, but some of her DHEA had cascaded into testosterone and caused her to have a higher testosterone level. Anxiety and irritability can be side effects of a testosterone level that is too high.

Randa's doctor suggested that she reduce the amount of DHEA she was taking from 25 to 10 milligrams a day and have a follow-up test in thirty days. Randa was ready to stop taking DHEA altogether. She was surprised and alarmed to learn that her testosterone level had risen. But after she and her doctor talked more about using saliva testing for measuring and monitoring her use of DHEA, she felt more comfortable. A month later, she was pleased to learn that her DHEA level was 150 pg/ml. What's more, her testosterone level had fallen to 38 pg/ml, well within the target range for a woman her age. Randa was feeling like her energetic and happy self again.

FRIEDA'S STORY

A 56-year-old widow who had recently remarried, Frieda was experiencing low libido and had been seeing headlines about testosterone's ability to reignite a postmenopausal woman's sexual spark. She asked her doctor if testosterone might help her to feel more interested in lovemaking again. Fortunately for Frieda, her doctor wasn't ready to take that step without more information. He wanted to test all of her hormone levels and do a Dpd test so he could have a complete picture of her hormonal profile.

Frieda's baseline saliva test showed low estrogen and progesterone levels, but the amount of DHEA, testosterone, and cortisol that her body was producing was fine. Her Dpd, however, came back elevated.

Frieda was concerned about the results of her Dpd test. Like Lana, she had recently had a normal DEXA scan, so she, too, was confused. Frieda's doctor used the analogy of a smoke detector to help her better understand her test results. Smoke detectors today have early-warning buzzers that tell you when the battery is running low. This enables you to be sure your detector is always in working order. Dpd can work like an early-warning signal, too: It can tell you when your rate of bone loss begins to increase. This enables you to take steps to intervene before any real loss has occurred.

Balancing Frieda's progesterone and estrogen levels with a 300-milligram sustained-release progesterone tablet and a 0.1-milligram weekly estradiol patch restored her libido, and she and her new husband were very happy. Had Frieda's doctor prescribed the testosterone without first testing her, Frieda might have had an unwanted increase in her testosterone level because it was not testosterone she needed. Supplemental testosterone might have produced unwanted side effects like Randa's, but Frieda didn't have to worry about that because her saliva test revealed precisely what hormones she needed. Every woman is unique. Symptoms that might indicate a need for testosterone in one person may be the result of a deficiency of something else in another.

THERE ARE MANY ways to take HRT. You can take old-fashioned HRT, with its one-size-fits-all doses of synthetic and animal-derived hormones. You can have a blood test first, or no test at all. You can buy natural hormones over the counter and take them on your own as well. But if you settle for any of those approaches, you will be missing out on individualized and customized hormone replacement therapy with solutions that are designed especially for you.

Along with saliva testing, assessment of your risk factors, your current health, and your family health history are all important factors in deciding whether you should take HRT and, if so, what you should take and when. They provide important information that is helpful in formulating your individualized hormone replacement therapy program. And they are critical tools in the diagnosis, treatment, and management of chronic degenerative diseases.

We believe that every woman should be able to benefit from all the new options there are for health and longevity. We want to inspire you to become an active participant in your health care and your hormone care. In the chapter that follows, we will prepare you to discuss individualized hormone replacement therapy with your doctor.

12

GETTING STARTED

Managed care now dominates health care in the United States. It is designed to maximize the efficiency of both health-care providers and health-care facilities. As a result of this new approach to medicine, many doctors are busier. They have tighter schedules. Some of them are even required to see a certain number of patients each day. In the good old days of house calls and leisurely office visits, doctors had more time to spend with you. Now, many of us feel we do not have the same connection with our doctors that we remember having when we were younger. As patients, sometimes we feel like we get lost in the shuffle. We feel like we have to fend for ourselves, figure things out on our own. And in reality, sometimes we do. But all of these changes aren't necessarily bad. They actually may give us the opportunity to become more involved in our own health care.

Before managed care, doctors had not only more time to spend with each patient but also more time to keep up with all of the innovations in health care. Pharmaceutical sales representatives used to schedule appointments with doctors to inform them of the latest advances in medications. That has changed, too. In an effort to find new ways of getting information to doctors, pharmaceutical manufacturers have recognized the value of consumer education. You may have noticed that in many of your favorite magazines and on television, pharmaceutical companies now advertise their new drug therapies directly to potential consumers. Right after an advertisement for a high-tech computer or a fast new car, you are likely to encounter an ad for an allergy or heart medication. The ad tells you what the medication is for, how effective it is, and how much better you are going to feel after you take it.

These advertisements are simple but potent. This powerful new educational tool is affecting the practice of medicine. A patient can go to her doctor, talk about the medication or therapy she has just read about, and ask to have it prescribed. In essence, patients are now bringing solutions to their doctors—in some cases, solutions their doctors may not have been aware of.

For many women, hormone replacement is vitally important, if not necessary, for their continued health and well-being. Yet most doctors are not as experienced with this complex and rapidly expanding branch of medicine as they would like to be. Many doctors we have talked to are increasingly frustrated with their situation. Because more and more women are entering menopause (more than 1.5 million American women a year, or approximately 4,300 a day, at the current rate), doctors want to be able to serve their patients in the best way they can. You may be fortunate enough to have a doctor who prides him- or herself in keeping as current as possible on all issues related to women's health and hormone replacement. He or she may already know about saliva testing, compounding and titrating hormones, and monitoring HRT. This is a best-case scenario. If this is the kind of doctor you have, just making an appointment to discuss whether you are a candidate for HRT may be all you have to do.

But you may have a doctor who has an incredibly heavy workload and no time to investigate all the new options available for HRT. Most doctors don't have the time to keep up with all the research that is constantly emerging. Consequently, your doctor may not be familiar with individualizing and monitoring hormone replacement. And if your doctor is not familiar with these techniques, he or she may be unwilling to try them.

Whatever the dynamics of your relationship with your doctor, we are going to help you make some decisions about what is right for you and then take action to ensure that you get what you want. This may be as simple as scheduling an appointment or as challenging, yet rewarding, as engaging in a spirited dialogue with your doctor. In this chapter, we will guide you through the process of meeting with your doctor and telling him or her what you have learned in this book. We will prepare you for the challenges you may encounter if you meet with a doctor who is unfamiliar with this new approach to HRT. We want to give you all the information you need to feel confident in your knowledge about individualized hormone replacement and to ask for the best hormone replacement treatments available. We would like you to feel enthusiastic about what you have learned; certain in your opinion that if you need HRT, you want it customized to suit your needs; and confident of your ability to discuss this with your doctor. Finally, recognizing the reality of health care in the United States today, we will address the issue of dealing with your health-insurance provider so you will know what your options are if this treatment is not automatically covered by your plan.

BECOMING AN ACTIVE PARTICIPANT

There are three important parts to becoming an active participant in your own health care: you, your doctor, and your health-insurance plan. We would like you to take a moment and give some thought to the kind of a patient you are, the kind of doctor you have, and how much you know about the type of insurance coverage you have.

Let's start with you. Maybe you are a patient who likes to take an active role, who is an active participant in your own health care. The idea of having a better understanding of how your body works and what it needs is exciting to you. You enjoy sharing new discoveries you have made on your own with your doctor, and you are not afraid to ask for the standard of care you want. We are going to give you some tools you can use to do just that. If, on the other hand, you usually rely on your doctor to tell you what you need, this could be a little more challenging for you. But think about it this way: Changing roles with your doctor— becoming the provider rather than the recipient of information—could give you the opportunity to share something important with him or her, something that not only will help you but also may help all of your doctor's other female patients as well. Keep in mind that you will be providing a service to your doctor when you share what you have learned from this book. By stressing the importance of individualizing hormone replacement, you are telling your doctor how important it is to you that you be treated as an individual.

If you encounter skepticism from your doctor, we don't want you to let your enthusiasm be dampened by it. Your hormonal balance has a powerful influence over your life. Maintaining this balance in the manner that is specific to you is crucial. As we have seen, all of your hormones work together. If one of them is out of sync, all the others can be affected. Having your health care tailored to you rather than being subjected to a general one-size-fits-all approach is really a higher form of medical treatment. You deserve the best medical care there is, and you are simply asking your doctor to be the best that he or she can be.

In order to talk to your doctor about hormones, it isn't necessary to engage in a complicated or technical medical discussion. Talking about your own health care from a personal point of view is very effective. Address your needs, express your concerns, and share what you have learned in language that is comfortable and familiar to you. You don't need to compete with anyone to get your point across. You know what you want, and you have a right to ask for it.

Once you bring up the subject of this new approach to hormone replacement, you may find you have a doctor who says, "I'm intrigued. I'd like more information." More and more doctors want to know about natural hormones and how to prescribe them as effectively as possible. In most cases, as soon as physicians are introduced to saliva testing and dose individualizing, they realize it takes the guesswork out of hormone replacement.

WORKING WITH YOUR DOCTOR

Now let us pay a visit to the doctor's office and work through some of the actual situations and conversations you may face when you approach your doctor about this program. Let's suppose you are just beginning to suspect that you may be a candidate for hormone replacement. You've been having hot flashes, your sleep pattern seems to be getting worse every day, you feel a little fuzzy-headed, sex is out, and "Cry Me a

River" seems to be your new favorite song. You suspect that you might need hormone therapy. Now that you have read this book, you want to be sure before you start taking anything that it's exactly what you need.

Asking for What You Want

When you arrive for your doctor's appointment, you tell him what you have been experiencing. He understands completely. "It's menopause," he says, as he pulls out his prescription pad and scribbles something down.

"What's that?" you want to know.

"Premarin and Provera," he responds. "It will do the trick."

This is exactly what most women experience in their doctors' offices today as they enter menopause. And it is the perfect opportunity to begin a dialogue with your doctor about why you would like to explore other options. The following are the main issues you will want to address with your doctor:

- You want to use natural, replacement hormones because they match the ones your body produces.
- Before you take anything, you want to have your saliva hormone levels tested so that you will know what your free-hormone levels are and what you need.
- You want the doses of any hormones you take to be individualized so they are just right for you.
- You want to work with your doctor in monitoring your free-hormone levels throughout treatment to make sure your therapy is working for you.

Be prepared for the fact that your doctor may insist that equine estrogen (such as Premarin) and synthetic progestin (Provera) are the norm. Remember that physicians get used to using certain medications. They become familiar with them and therefore feel comfortable prescribing them. You can respond by saying simply, "I don't want to take them because they do not match the hormones that my body makes for itself. There can be side effects with those drugs, and I would like to avoid them."

Your doctor may counter this by telling you, "These hormones are the ones we know the most about," and he or she may try to reassure you that you will feel better and that they will protect you against osteoporosis. You can then let your doctor know that you are aware of the studies that have been done on these hormone products and that you know they show that replacement therapy is beneficial. But you also know that it is estradiol that is so beneficial, and that equine estrogen is horse estrogen, unique to horses and not identical to what your body makes. You would prefer taking 100 percent natural, identical-to-human estradiol over horse estrogen any day.

Most doctors know there is a difference between synthetic or animal-derived hormones and natural hormones. What they may not know is how to prescribe natural hormones. If your doctor is not convinced and suggests that he or she does not really have enough information on the dosing of natural hormones, you can help by telling him or her that there are pharmacists who specialize in individualizing hormone replacement and that they will be able to assist.

Regarding Provera—and many doctors automatically prescribe Provera with Premarin—your response may have to be a little different. Progesterone is the body's natural estrogen balancer, but remember that Provera is a synthetic progestin—a molecule that does not match your body's own progesterone. The Postmenopausal Estrogen/Progestin Interventions (PEPI) study helped us to identify the differences between natural progesterone and synthetic progestins in preserving a beneficial lipid profile (see page 57). Progesterone has a positive effect on HDL ("good") cholesterol, but progestins do not. In fact, whereas progesterone elevates HDL, progestins lower it. Maintaining a healthy lipid profile is a very important aspect of caring for your heart.

If you mention the PEPI study, your doctor may say, "Oh yes, the PEPI study . . ." But he or she may not remember what the results of the study were, especially if he or she is not completely familiar with this area of medicine. Every doctor who is treating women today should know about this study. You can do your doctor a great service if you can summarize its important points. (Your local librarian may be able to help you locate a copy of the study.) Remind your doctor that the PEPI study found that when natural replacement progesterone is combined with estrogen, it provides better cardiovascular protection than synthetic progestins do. The PEPI study also found that women who take replacement hormones after menopause tend to gain less weight than women who don't take them. You can remind your doctor that studies suggest that natural progesterone may have a protective effect on breast tissue and that

progesterone protects the endometrium (uterine lining). There are studies that support the effectiveness of natural progesterone, whether taken
orally or administered transdermally. Synthetic progestins do not have all
of these benefits. That's quite a case for natural progesterone, and that's
what you want to take.

If you have had a hysterectomy, your doctor might tell you that since
you no longer have your uterus, you don't need progesterone, because
you don't need any protection against endometrial cancer. But remember, progesterone works throughout your body. Taking supplemental
progesterone may help maintain your bones, protect your breast tissue,
and maintain the proper balance among all of your other sex steroid hormones, including DHEA and testosterone. These are substantial benefits.
While not all of the benefits cited here have yet been confirmed, existing data do suggest that there are many reasons to have progesterone prescribed with estradiol. In fact, it is our position that you really wouldn't
want to take estradiol without progesterone, whether you have a uterus
or not. After all, nature designed estrogen and progesterone to work together in your body.

Meeting Resistance

In spite of all this information, your doctor may still be convinced that,
when you use Premarin and Provera together, they work in a certain way
and that there is no way you can substitute natural replacement hormones and get the same results. Many doctors feel this way, and in many
ways it is understandable, but more and more studies are being done
every day, and we have more clinical experience every year to prove that
when you use natural replacement hormones, you get better results.

In support of these findings, you might want to remind your doctor
that major pharmaceutical companies are now developing natural replacement hormone products because they recognize the benefits of
these formulas over synthetics. Estrace, Climara, Vivelle, and Estraderm
are all natural estradiol products. Prometrium is a natural progesterone
product. When you mention this, your doctor may say he or she is willing to prescribe one of these products for you, but remember, though
their formulas are identical to human hormones, these products come
only in standard doses, so they do not take your individual needs into account. Prometrium, for example, comes in a 100-milligram dose. For

some women, this might be just fine, but for others it will be either too high or too low.

If you tell your physician that you would like to know what your hormone levels are before you take any prescription medication, he or she may respond by telling you, "It's not necessary to do a test because your menstrual cycles have stopped and you are having lots of symptoms. Your hormones are just naturally going to be low." Or he or she may respond by saying, "Fine. I'll order a blood test." In either case, this is the time to tell your doctor that you want your free-hormone levels tested in saliva. And you don't want only estrogen and progesterone tested—you want to know where your DHEA, testosterone, and cortisol levels stand, too, and what your rate of bone metabolism is. If your doctor looks a little surprised at this point, you might want to take a deep breath and tell him or her what you have learned about free and bound hormones (see Chapter 2).

Then you can explain that you want a more complete picture of where you stand, hormonally, than one based on your symptoms alone. You want to know exactly what's going on with your hormones—which are high, which are low, and which are right where they should be. Point out that if you are going to consider taking HRT, you want to maximize its health benefits by taking all your sex steroid hormones into account. You want to bring them all into balance, within the range that will provide the greatest health benefit, relief of symptoms, and protection against disease.

Individualizing hormone replacement therapy is an art. You can explain to your doctor that another reason you want to do saliva testing and monitoring is to find out exactly how you are responding to therapy and whether you need any adjustments. You can refer your doctor to the information in the back of this book for resources and assistance in prescribing an HRT program that is tailor-made for you.

Don't be afraid to tell your doctor that if you are going to take hormones, you want to have as much information as possible. You know there have been risks associated with HRT, and you want to minimize them, and you also want to know whether the therapy is working. If you are going to take HRT to protect you from osteoporosis, then you want to know that you are in fact being protected.

A doctor may believe that he or she is satisfying a patient's desire to take something natural by prescribing natural hormones, but if he or she doesn't test and titrate the dosage, then the patient's hormone replacement program is not really individualized just for her. Recent tests have shown that low doses of natural estradiol do in fact raise estradiol levels sufficiently for many women and provide protection against degenerative disease. The standard dose of Premarin is 0.625 milligrams. A recent study demonstrated that significantly less than that dose of natural estradiol (in 0.03-milligram patches) did indeed provide protection against osteoporosis.

You may find that your doctor is unfamiliar with the Dpd test. In this case, you will want to explain that it is a bone-resorption test. It is a diagnostic tool that will enable your doctor to monitor your bone health and how your therapy is working for you. A customized hormone replacement program goes well beyond any one of its single elements. It is the combination of saliva testing, bone-resorption evaluation, dose individualization, and monitoring that makes such a program truly individualized. Each element is as important as any of the others. Each works in its own specific ways, and, just like your hormones, they all work together to give you the most comprehensive and rational hormone management program there is.

Don't be discouraged if at first you are not successful in a dialogue with your doctor. And, by all means, don't give up. Just because your doctor may not be open to something new, there are others who are. There are many physicians who use individualized hormone restoration. You may want to get a referral and consult with someone else. In more cases than not, though, doctors seem to be very happy to learn about this new way of prescribing HRT. We urge you not to be afraid to bring it up and not to assume that your doctor knows about it.

Your doctor may say, "Well, fine, I do think these natural hormones are a reasonable alternative, but the saliva test has not been proven." You can tell him or her that there are thirty years of experience that say, yes, saliva testing *has* been proven to be an accurate and precise way of determining free-hormone levels. And remind your doctor that medicine is constantly changing. We are continually learning more about our bodies and our environment. In many cases, what we once thought was safe has turned out, after years of examination, not to be. For over thirty years, doctors have been prescribing synthetic versions of hormones in one-size-fits-all doses. There is a great deal of evidence now that it may not be in our best interest to continue doing it that way.

UNDERSTANDING YOUR MEDICAL PLAN

Many of us take for granted that our health-insurance plans cover our best interests. In some cases this is true, but in many cases it is not. This is a perfect opportunity to really explore your health-insurance plan. Read your handbook—get to know all the ins and outs of it. You may be covered for some procedures and not even know it, while you may assume you are covered for others but in reality are not. Understanding your health-insurance plan lets you know exactly what kind of medical treatment you can expect to receive.

Many patients assume that their doctors know what is covered by their insurance. Sometimes they do, but often they don't. When you encounter resistance from a doctor, that may be precisely what he or she is concerned about—doing a procedure, ordering a test, or prescribing a medication that isn't going to be covered. If you are informed about your own policy, it will help you in your discussion with your doctor.

There are many different kinds of health insurance. Each has its own criteria for what it covers and what it does not. You may have the kind of insurance plan that allows you to be a freelance patient, which means you can select your doctor based on your needs. In this type of situation, your doctor generally has the freedom to make decisions about your treatment based on what he or she feels is appropriate for you. In other words, your doctor can prescribe what he or she feels is necessary. Or you may have the kind of plan that provides you with a list of network doctors from which you must choose your primary-care physician. Network doctors may have some restrictions on what they can prescribe for you and may have to provide you with a referral in order for you to see a specialist.

Then, too, some insurance plans provide coverage for prescription medications, and you can fill your prescriptions wherever you choose. Others require you to fill your prescriptions within a particular HMO system. Finally, there are some insurance plans that restrict doctors to prescribing only certain medications. In other words, your doctor may want to prescribe an individualized dose of natural progesterone for you but is not allowed to prescribe anything other than Provera. Having a full understanding of your insurance coverage before you begin your discussion with your doctor will help you better understand its assets and limitations.

In much the same way that you may have to choose your physician from within your insurance network, you may also be required to use only a selected testing laboratory and be limited to a specific group of testing procedures. Many insurance plans want you to stay as much within their system as possible. If you are in an insurance group that covers only certain medications and procedures, your doctor may still be willing to prescribe what you prefer, but you may have to pay for the tests and the hormone prescriptions yourself.

If you belong to a health plan that tells you it doesn't cover individualized hormone therapy and monitoring, don't be discouraged. Your doctor can write a letter of medical necessity to your insurance company. This is a letter written on your behalf certifying that the type of care you need is not available within the existing scope of the plan, so you require special consideration. Many doctors who work in managed-care settings are excited about this new approach to HRT. They recognize the need for more effective and safer forms of hormone replacement, and many offer to write letters of medical necessity in an attempt to have an individualized and customized hormone replacement program covered within their medical groups (see the Appendix for an example of this kind of letter). Another approach you can take is to write your own letter to your insurance company explaining why you want to pursue this treatment program. In such a letter, you would approach your insurance company in much the same way you would a doctor who is unfamiliar with individualized HRT. You would become your own advocate.

Whether you are independently insured or a member of an HMO, as a first course of action you may want to consider taking this book to your doctor. The suggestions and summaries of studies it contains may appeal to your doctor and demonstrate to him or her the value of (and the research behind) individualized hormone therapy using natural replacement hormones and ongoing monitoring of free-hormone levels. This could motivate your doctor to approach the health-management company he or she is affiliated with and suggest that this become one of the hormone replacement protocols it covers.

Remember, the better you understand yourself, your doctor, and your insurance coverage, the more likely you are to be successful in having what you want prescribed for you and in being reimbursed by your medical insurance plan for it. Of course, if your doctor is willing to prescribe it for you, and your insurance company absolutely will not cover it, you can accept your doctor's prescription and pay for the program yourself. For most people, the cost is quite reasonable, especially when you consider how much benefit you can derive from it.

THE IMPORTANCE OF YOU

It is important to have as much information as you can about yourself as you begin a hormone replacement program. You do not want to take anything you don't need. You don't want to take more of anything than you need. And you certainly want to make sure that if you are taking hormones, you are taking a dosage that provides you with the benefits that are your very reason for taking them. Each aspect of the program is equally as important.

More than 50 million women are currently in menopause. Many of them are concerned about taking hormones. Most women don't want to take synthetic drugs. If there is a better, more natural alternative, they want to be given the opportunity to choose it. More and more women are going to their doctors and asking them to prescribe natural replacement hormones.

Hormone replacement therapy is a young science, and researchers are constantly expanding their knowledge of it. Every day we are learning more. We still have a long way to go before we completely understand all the complexities of the endocrine system, but one thing we do know is what you have learned from this book: Your hormonal balance is delicate, intricate, and uniquely your own.

Hormone restoration has never before been done this way. But soon it won't be done any other way. It has never been better, safer, or more rational. We want to change the way hormones are prescribed, and we want you to know what all your choices are when it comes to HRT, because we want you to have the best that medicine has to offer so that you can be the best that you can be.

EPILOGUE:
THE FUTURE OF HRT

Science and medicine are making dramatic breakthroughs every day in our understanding of how hormones work in the body and the role they play in keeping us healthy. Hormone replacement therapy has opened the door to a bold new world of anti-aging medicine, which is now a rapidly expanding and evolving area of science. Thanks to all the research being done, we are continually learning more about the miracle of hormones. There are countless research studies in progress now, and many new developments in longevity and rejuvenation are just ahead on the horizon. Some of the most exciting areas under investigation are the circadian-rhythm hormones cortisol and melatonin; sex steroid hormones and the brain; testosterone replacement for women; hormone replacement for men; phytohormones; alpha and beta hormone receptors; selective estrogen receptor modulators (SERMS); and super hormone cocktails.

Stress has become an ever-increasing part of our daily lives. The fast pace of life made possible by modern technology has led to many exciting changes and innovations in our lifestyles. In some ways, life has become easier; in others ways, it seems we are constantly being challenged to do more, learn more, remember more, even succeed more. Consequently, we are under more stress than ever before. As a result, there is an enormous amount of research being done on cortisol, the stress hormone.

The more science learns about stress, the more it confirms the damaging effects that too much cortisol can have on our health. For example, elevated cortisol levels can make the implantation of a fertilized egg less likely. Lowering or managing cortisol levels may therefore have a very positive effect on women who are having difficulty conceiving. Learning more about stress management and developing effective ways to control this important hormone are essential.

Using new imaging techniques, scientists have found that the high cortisol levels that come with chronic stress can actually damage and shrink the brain. Excessive cortisol has been associated with atrophy of the hippocampus—as much as 25 percent. The hippocampus, or learning center of the brain, is used for processing and storing information. It is also responsible for regulating your hormonal stress response—releasing stress hormones when you need them and shutting off the release when stress has subsided. Damage to the hippocampus can result in an inability to turn off the stress response, which in turn keeps cortisol levels elevated and sets in motion a very destructive cycle. Losing a quarter of your hippocampus can also mean substantial losses in cognitive function and emotional well-being. Studies have shown that women who suffer chronic depression and stress develop significant atrophy of the hippocampus. Newborns who suffer great stress just after birth also show mental impairment, including memory deficits. Salivary cortisol levels in airline pilots and cabin crew exposed to continual jet lag have been found to be much higher after long flights than those of shorter distances. Their higher cortisol levels also were associated with cognitive deficits.

Interestingly, chronic insomnia increases levels of cortisol. Insomniacs secrete high levels of cortisol in the evening and nighttime hours, when cortisol levels should be low. This means that they are producing stress-hormone levels that actually prevent them from sleeping. Sustained, round-the-clock activation of the body's stress response system combined with too little sleep can aggravate and intensify other medical conditions like high blood pressure and digestive disorders, and weaken the body's ability to fight off illness.

Hypertension or a family history of heart disease can lead to an exaggerated blood-pressure response to mental stress. In one study, women with this profile who were on HRT, however, did not have the same elevated blood-pressure response when confronted with a stressful situation. Conversely, women who had the same risk factors but who were not taking hormones, who experienced rage fairly regularly in response to stress, demonstrated three times the increase in blood pressure as their HRT-using counterparts.

More research is being done on the effects of hormonal changes on circadian rhythms. Melatonin is a hormone produced in the pineal gland and is mainly known for its role in the sleep/wake cycle. Melatonin production is affected by the amount of bright light you are exposed to before you go to bed, the amount of alcohol you drink on a regular basis, how old you are, and where you are on your hormonal river of life. Optimum melatonin levels are produced when you have a balanced exposure to daylight and darkness. As the sun goes down and darkness falls, melatonin production goes up. It helps you to fall asleep and stay asleep. However, research is showing us that melatonin also helps to regulate a number of other biological processes besides sleep, including mood, reproduction, tumor growth, degenerative brain disease, and aging.

Two important studies done at the Fred Hutchinson Cancer Research Center in Seattle and at the Harvard Medical Center have discovered that women who work swing and graveyard shifts appear to be at higher risk for breast cancer than women who do not. This may be due to their increased exposure to artificial light at night and decreased exposure to sunlight during the day. Some scientists believe this is a key element in breast-cancer research. Animal studies have shown that melatonin can inhibit the growth of breast-cancer tumors. There is mounting evidence that melatonin may stimulate immunity. A potent antioxidant, melatonin can permeate cells in the body and protect them from free-radical damage. Animal studies have shown that it can protect delicate brains cells from damage as well.

Brain research is one of the most exciting frontiers in science. The development of new technologies allows us to view the brain in ways not previously available, yielding exciting new insights into the relationship between hormones and brain function. An enormous body of scientific research now demonstrates that estrogen is essential for optimal brain function. It seems to promote and protect the growth and viability of neurons (brain cells) and dendrites (the connections brain cells use to communicate with one another). Estrogen also protects blood vessels from plaque formation and increases blood flow throughout the brain. The flow of blood throughout the brain is what fuels the brain with the nutrients and oxygen it needs to thrive. Protection against Alzheimer's disease may be one of estrogen's most important functions.

Not only are hot flashes uncomfortable, but we now know that they also may be harmful to the brain. Nearly 85 percent of menopausal women experience hot flashes at some time or another, some mild, some much more serious. Using a noninvasive imaging technique called single-photon computed tomography (SPECT), researchers found that women who had low estrogen levels had decreased blood flow throughout the brain even when they were cool and calm. During a hot flash, blood flow became even more compromised. Worse yet, the vascular changes seen in these women were the same as those in people with mild to moderate Alzheimer's disease. Estrogen is hard to beat for relieving hot flashes.

Estrogen also influences the production and concentration of key mood-enhancing chemicals in the brain, such as serotonin and the endorphins. Millions of people suffer from depression, and women are twice as likely as men to experience a serious depression at some time in their lives. Such women are often given antidepressants when in reality it is possible that an evaluation of their hormone levels could reveal the true, hormonal cause of their blue moods.

But estrogen doesn't work alone in the brain. New studies are looking at the role of DHEA, progesterone, and testosterone in brain function. Testosterone is being shown to be a powerful mood-enhancing hormone able not only to lift a woman's spirits but also to restore her self-confidence and sense of well-being. Studies of aging men have shown that the higher their testosterone levels, the better they score on cognitive tests. While the same cognitive data are not available for women, it may be that testosterone is as important to the functioning of women's brains as it is to men's. More and more studies are revealing the critical role testosterone plays in all areas of women's health.

Traditional hormone replacement for women has consisted mainly of estrogen and progesterone. However, new findings suggest that testosterone may be a welcome addition to a woman's replacement therapy. Recently hailed for its ability to reignite a woman's libido and restore her desire for sex, testosterone's role in a woman's overall health may be more far-reaching than was ever believed. In women, in addition to enhancing mood and a sense of well-being, testosterone replacement may relieve depression, rejuvenate energy, help to build lean body mass, and protect her bones, brain, and heart.

Men, too, are becoming interested in hormone replacement therapy, particularly in testosterone, DHEA, and androstenedione supplementation. And we are finding that hormone restoration may have as many positive and far-reaching benefits for men as it does for women. Just as hormone supplementation affects a woman's hormone levels, it affects a man's hormonal profile, too. It is as important for men to know what their hormone levels are as it is for women and to evaluate the influence that supplementation has on those levels.

Recent studies have shown that increasing testosterone levels in men can relieve many symptoms associated with aging—decreased libido, lack of energy, decreased strength and/or endurance, loss of muscle mass, feelings of sadness or irritability, and sexual dysfunction. Salivary hormone-level tests that reveal low testosterone can help a physician to determine whether or not a man is suffering from hypogonadism, a syndrome characterized by decreases in erectile function, libido, muscle mass and strength, and bone density. This is an important advance in men's health care. Maybe Viagra isn't a man's only option—or even the best one. In fact, the rush to rely on an anti-impotence drug for sexual dysfunction may be not only premature but inadequate as well. Sexual dysfunction in men encompasses more than one symptom. Testosterone replacement may be a more comprehensive approach and certainly a more natural one.

Androstenedione is an androgen that is a precursor to testosterone. It is now being sold over the counter as a nutritional supplement and has been getting a great deal of press. Studies have shown that supplemental androstenedione does have the potential to cascade in the body and influence testosterone and DHEA levels. This could be an important finding, because we know that there is a definite relationship between male potency and testosterone.

Androgens also play an important role in hair loss in both men and women. The cycle of hair growth is controlled by an enzyme called *5 alpha-reductase type 2,* which converts testosterone into dihydrotestosterone (DHT). DHT is the active form of testosterone and is present in both men and women. Studies have shown that DHT plays an important role in hair loss. Blocking the formation of DHT allows hair follicles that are inactive to become active again and make new hairs. In women, estrogen seems to help block the formation of DHT. As a woman ages, however, and her estrogen levels decline, her DHT levels can begin to climb. Estrogen replacement may help to keep DHT levels down. Though men are not candidates for estrogen replacement, initial studies indicate that progesterone may be an effective 5-alpha-reductase inhibitor that can block the production of DHT.

Phytohormones (plant hormones), particularly the isoflavones, are also generating a great deal of excitement in the scientific community. Isoflavones are plant estrogens found in legumes such as soybeans. It appears that these phytoestrogens have estrogenic effects in the body and may act as surrogates for our own hormones. They may function in a way very similar to natural hormones. This is an important area of research. Studies have already demonstrated that eating soy foods can decrease levels of cholesterol, low-density lipoproteins (LDLs), and triglycerides. Animal studies have shown that the isoflavones have a beneficial effect on some cancers. And isoflavones have been shown to work as potent antioxidants and free-radical scavengers.

Even though more is being revealed about phytoestrogens every day, we still don't know precisely what role they might play in hormone restoration. There is still so much to learn about them. Do they actually mimic our own hormones? Or do the benefits they seem to offer come from other valuable nutritional components they possess that we don't completely understand yet? The answers are not all in.

Hormone receptors are another hot area of scientific investigation. The recent discovery of different types of estrogen and progesterone receptors is expanding the parameters of hormone science. Estrogen α and β receptors and progesterone A and B receptors are showing us that hormone receptors may be as complex as hormones themselves. The role these different types of receptors play in the hormonal activity that goes on in the body is not yet fully understood. However, it is known that each type of receptor allows its hormone to convey different messages to tissues and cells. In effect, these receptors broaden the reach of the hormone by increasing the repertoire of functions it has. Knowledge of these subgroups of hormone receptors is furthering our understanding of why hormones have such diverse actions in the various tissues throughout the body. This research has already led to the development of products such as selective estrogen receptor modulators (SERMS), or "designer estrogens," as some people call them.

Women are using SERMs such as raloxifene (Evista) as alternatives to the standard replacement estrogens. SERMS turn on only certain estrogen responses in the body and block others. Through a very complex biochemical process, SERMs interact with receptor cells in the bones and heart, but not with receptors in the uterus or breast. It has been proposed that they may provide the benefits of estrogen's bone and heart protection without any of the risks associated with synthetic or animal-derived conventional estrogen replacement. But are they able to confer the same benefits that natural, identical-to-human hormones provide? Does the body recognize them as its own? Maybe SERMs do offer some protection against endometrial hyperplasia and breast disease, but do they offer enough protection overall? For example, what about estrogen's important role in brain health?

We don't yet know how SERMs interact, if they do at all, with estrogen receptors in the brain. This is an important area of research because studies have now shown that estrogen increases the production of serotonin. Serotonin is a chemical produced in the brain that affects mood. If you don't have enough serotonin, depression can set in. There is a great deal of controversy over whether this selective-receptor interaction is what the body needs. Interacting with only some estrogen receptors and not others is not a natural, balanced process. Many questions still remain concerning the inability of SERMs to interact with your receptors in the same balanced way that both your own hormones and natural replacement hormones do.

Super hormone cocktails. What are they? These convenient-to-use, often potent hormone combination formulas are being touted as powerful anti-aging medicine. Taking hormones in combination form can provide hormones to your body in a way that mimics what your body provides for itself. But individual dosages and monitoring of responses are important factors in any form of HRT. Given what we know about how powerful hormones are, it is important to remember that a little goes a long way and that more is not necessarily better. If you are going to take a super hormone cocktail, it would be best to take one that has been formulated especially to meet your individual needs.

Combination therapies are an important area of investigation for another reason. A decline in the level of one hormone may not be a singular event. In fact, a decline—or, for that matter, an increase—in the level of one hormone can affect the balance among all of your sex steroid hormones. Science is vigorously investigating the importance of hormone ratios.

The pharmaceutical industry is exploding with new options for HRT. Pharmaceutical companies are clamoring to bring new natural replacement formulations and combination hormone-delivery systems to the marketplace. Patches are being formulated not only in lower and lower dosage amounts but also in combination formulas. Choices abound. But even as our options expand, individualizing, customizing, and monitoring any hormone therapy are still the keys. As more products become available, more research has to be done on individual variability. No one answer is or will be right for everyone.

The importance of assessing hormone levels before midlife is another area of investigation. Knowing what your hormone levels are when you are in your thirties could be important if you decide to begin hormone restoration therapy later in life. In the same way that a baseline bone-density scan or mammogram provides an important frame of reference, knowing what your hormone levels are when you are in the peak of hormonal health could serve as a guideline for optimal restoration levels.

Hormones are revolutionizing medicine. They are important to our health, and they influence every aspect of our lives. And there are still so many unanswered questions about them. The only way we will be able to answer them all is if we continue to strive toward a more comprehensive understanding of the hundreds of hormone interactions that go on in our bodies every day.

The study of elderly Americans being conducted by the New England Centenarian Group is providing many new insights into how we age. Did you know that women who have babies naturally when they are over forty are four times as likely to reach the age of 100 than women who have babies when they are younger? This is not because childbearing promotes long life. It is because older mothers appear to have reproductive systems that are aging more slowly. This raises many important questions about the significant role optimal hormone levels may play in how and when we age. Currently, 50,000 Americans are centenarians, and 80 percent of them are women. Our aging population is and will continue to provide a fascinating and important area of scientific investigation.

There are currently nearly 90 million women between the ages of twenty and sixty. There are 70 million Americans over the age of fifty, more than half of them women. Soon there will be more Americans over fifty years of age than under eighteen. By the year 2020, nearly 50 million women will be over the age of fifty-five. The baby boomers have reached midlife and brought with them a growing demand for ways to feel better, look better, and live longer.

More and more doctors are being faced with all the complexities of hormone replacement therapy. And they are recognizing the importance of individualized natural hormone replacement programs. They are seeking a better understanding of the different hormone-delivery systems and learning how to adjust doses in order to minimize side effects and maximize therapeutic effectiveness. Continuing medical education courses are now being offered by a variety of sources to help physicians better understand all the nuances of individualized natural hormone replacement therapy. Treating patients as individuals is a more rational, proactive approach to HRT that allows doctors to address the hormonal needs of a rapidly expanding population of older patients in a much more effective way.

In order to answer all the questions we still have about hormones, science must remain committed to a continuing effort to unravel their mysteries. They are one of the most potent tools we have in our scientific investigation of how to remain healthy as we age. There seems to be no end to what we can learn in the coming decades about aging, longevity, and rejuvenation through the study of hormones.

Appendix:
Letter of Medical Necessity

Many insurance companies cover some or all of the procedures used in an individualized natural hormone replacement program. Some do not, however. If you are a member of a health-maintenance organization (HMO) or preferred-provider organization (PPO), it is important to go over your plan or discuss it with your benefits administrator.

In the event that your plan does not cover these services, it will be helpful to have your health-care provider establish that they are necessary by forwarding a letter of medical necessity to your insurance company. The following is a sample of the kind of letter your medical provider can submit on your behalf (substitute appropriate information for the items indicated in brackets).

SAMPLE LETTER OF MEDICAL NECESSITY FOR AN INDIVIDUALIZED NATURAL HORMONE REPLACEMENT PROGRAM

[Current date]
[Name and address of your insurance company]

Re: [Your name]
      [Your subscriber number]
      [Your diagnosis]
      [Your policy number]

Dear Sir or Madam:

I am writing on behalf of [your name] regarding my decision to begin her natural hormone replacement program in order to monitor and individualize her hormone replacement therapy. [Your physician can add more specific language regarding your condition here as appropriate.]

An individualized natural hormone replacement program protocol includes:

• Baseline saliva hormone-evaluation panel (estradiol, progesterone, testosterone, DHEA, cortisol).
• Urine deoxypyridinoline test to determine rate of bone resorption.
• Medication, titration, and dose adjustment to achieve desired therapeutic hormone levels (thirty-day post-therapy follow-up testing).
• Therapeutic intervention evaluation that includes hormone-level assessment and evaluation of bone-resorption rate after six to twelve months.

The initial diagnostic procedures of saliva testing and assessment of rate of bone loss, the individualized formulation of hormone prescription, and follow-up testing to evaluate response and progress were necessary for my patient. Below is a list of information about my patient's medical history, diagnosis, and treatment; a brief description of the assays; and my reason for ordering this program.

Patient History, Diagnosis, and Treatment

[Your name] is a [your age]-year-old woman with [your physician should insert information about your history, diagnosis, and current treatment regimen].

Diagnostic Assay Descriptions

1. Saliva Hormone Testing

A saliva hormone test uses highly specific antibodies (radioimmunoassay) to quantitate hormone levels. Determining and monitoring hormone levels in saliva provide a direct measure of the biologically active (free) fraction of steroid hormone present. Free hormone reflects the physiologically active component of total serum hormone. More than 90 percent of serum hormone is protein bound and therefore unavailable to the cells. By passive diffusion, only free (unbound) hormone enters saliva from serum. This is the same process by which hormones enter cells throughout the body.

Hormone levels have traditionally been assessed indirectly by using an FSH/LH test or directly by using a serum test. Serum tests generally measure only total hormone levels and do not accurately reflect free-hormone levels. The interaction between the sex steroids and FSH/LH levels is complex and cannot indicate hormone levels accurately. FSH and LH cannot be used to determine when hormone levels are too high in response to hormone replacement therapy (for dose-titration purposes).

Saliva testing provides a direct measure of the biologically active (free) fraction of steroid hormones present. Precise timing of sample collection facilitates the accurate measurement of peak and trough levels associated with HRT. Collecting saliva in the early A.M. permits the accurate assessment of diurnal hormones such as testosterone, cortisol, and DHEA. Precise timing within the menstrual cycle, if a woman is still cycling, can accurately pinpoint ovulatory and luteal hormone levels. Salivary steroid hormones are stable for up to three weeks at room temperature. Saliva hormone testing is noninvasive, economical, and more convenient than blood testing since the specimen can be collected at home at the appropriate time for analysis.

Studies demonstrate the accuracy of saliva for the measurement of free-hormone levels. Clinical trials have validated the specificity of this method by detecting increases and decreases in hormone levels following therapy.

2. Bone Metabolism Assessment

Until recently, urinary Dpd levels could be measured only by high-pressure liquid chromatography (HPLC). Now the Dpd assay can be performed by a simple, competitive-inhibition enzyme-linked immunosorbent assay (ELISA) performed on single first- or second-morning voids, or twenty-four-hour urine samples. Clinical studies have shown that this assay is highly sensitive and specific and superior to previously available assays for hydroxyproline and calcium excretion.

The Center of Medicare and Medicaid Services (CMS) mandates coverage and reimbursement by all Medicare carriers for testing requested by a licensed medical provider to:

1. Identify individuals with elevated bone resorption (loss) who have osteoporosis in whom response to treatment is being monitored.
2. Predict response (as assessed by bone-mass measurements) to FDA-approved antiresorptive therapy in postmenopausal women.

The Dpd assay is an accurate, quantitative tool for measuring urinary levels of deoxypyridinoline (Dpd), an important biochemical marker of the bone-resorption process. The assay enhances physicians' abilities to monitor the effects of antiresorptive drug and hormone therapies for patients with metabolic bone disease. Dpd is a cross-linking amino acid that is released as type I bone collagen degrades. The amount of this biochemical marker excreted in the urine directly reflects the bone-resorption rate. Clinical trials have validated the specificity of this marker by detecting an increase in its excretion in postmenopausal women and a decrease following antiresorptive therapies, such as HRT.

Traditionally, there has been no means to measure the direct effect of hormone replacement intervention on rate of bone resorption. Since there is an inverse relationship between rate of bone loss and increase in estrogen levels associated with HRT, periodic monitoring of this dynamic will provide a more comprehensive picture of a woman's response to therapy. Elevated Dpd results will be reevaluated in six- to twelve-month intervals in order to measure the effects of antiresorptive intervention such as hormone replacement.

The American Medical Association, American College of Clinical Endocrinology, American Society for Bone and Mineral Research, and the International Society for Clinical Densitometry have endorsed Dpd testing.

The American Association of Clinical Endocrinology Guidelines for Postmenopausal Osteoporosis states:

> Biochemical markers of bone turnover (loss of bone cells) may be useful for the following situations:
>
> 1. Assessing fracture risk in elder patients.
> 2. Assessing therapeutic responses to antiresorptive agents, such as estrogen and biphosphonates.
> 3. Identifying patients with high bone turnover (to predict rapid bone loss).
>
> The newer bone markers have been intensively studied for more than a decade. As a result, we can now confidently report their clinical utility in assessing risk for rapid bone loss and fracture, and monitoring therapy in postmenopausal women with or without osteoporosis.
>
> (Consensus of an Expert Panel cited in the *Journal of Densitometry* 2[3] [Fall 1999]: 323-342.)

Individualized Hormone Replacement Therapy

Individualized prescription therapy provides a woman with the proper dose of hormone replacement relative to her unique physiology. Reassessment of a woman's changing needs and her response to therapy allows for more effective treatment over time. An individualized natural hormone replacement program takes into consideration the diverse pharmacokinetics of replacement steroid hormones. After absorption, for example, some hormone preparations are metabolized substantially before they become available for systemic circulation. If a large amount of a hormone is metabolized on the first pass through the gut wall and the liver, then larger doses will be needed to achieve the same concentration.

Conversely, if hormone levels are too high, it might lead to immediate symptoms or, more important, the increased risk of breast cancer.

Factors that bear heavily on the efficacy of hormone replacement therapy are the half-life of the hormones, or the time required for the concentration of a drug to decline by 50 percent; the molecular structure of the replacement hormone; the amount of hormone administered and the amount being eliminated in a given time interval, which should lead to a steady-state concentration that recurs with each dose once equilibrium is achieved; the therapeutic range of concentrations associated with a high degree of efficacy and a low risk of dose-related toxicity; and the titration of dose to reach a balance between therapeutic and physiologic levels. All of these factors vary from patient to patient and require individual assessment.

Individualizing and monitoring hormone replacement therapy helps to avoid patient side effects resulting from excess dosing and therefore reduces the need for repeat office visits.

Rationale for Use of an Individualized Natural Hormone Replacement Program

The use of an individualized natural hormone replacement program was medically necessary because it is a responsive method of diagnosing and treating hormonal imbalance. This program is more precise and effective than other methods. [As appropriate, your physician should insert additional description of therapeutic decisions made based on your response to diagnosis and treatment.]

Attached are studies published in peer-reviewed medical journals that support the efficacy and clinical value of all aspects of this program.

Based on this letter and the attached materials, I believe that you will agree that the treatment was medically necessary and should be covered. I ask that you reconsider your prior decision and provide coverage and payment for this program.

Thank you for reviewing this case. If you require any additional information, please contact me at [your physician should insert his or her telephone number].

Sincerely,
[Your physician's name]

REFERENCES

American College of Obstetricians and Gynecologists, *Questions and Answers on Hormone Therapy: In Response to the Women's Health Initiative Study Results on Estrogen and Progestin Hormone Therapy* (Washington, D.C.: American College of Obstetricians and Gynecologists, August 2002).

W.C. Andrews, "Menopause," keynote address to the North America Menopause Society Annual Meeting, in *Menopause: The Journal of the North American Menopause Society* 2 (2) (1994): 59–65.

C.D. Arnaud, "Osteoporosis: Using 'Bone Markers' for Diagnosis and Monitoring," *Geriatrics* 51 (April 1996): 24–30.

G. Bachmann, J. Bancroft, G. Braunstein, et al., "Female Androgen Insufficiency: The Princeton Consensus Statement on Definition, Classification, and Assessment," *Fertility and Sterility* 77 (4) (April 2002): 660–665.

E. Barrett-Connor and D. Goodman-Gruen, "Prospective Study of Endogenous Sex Hormones and Fatal Cardiovascular Disease in Postmenopausal Women," *British Medical Journal* 311 (4 November 1995): 1193–1196.

E. Barrett-Connor, K.-T. Khaw, and S.S.C. Yen, "A Prospective Study of Dehydroepiandrosterone (DHEA) Sulfate, Mortality, and Cardiovascular Disease," *The New England Journal of Medicine* 315 (1986): 1519–1524.

N. Beckman, "Phyto-oestrogens and Compounds That Effect Oestrogen Metabolism—Parts I and II," *Australian Journal of Medical Herbalism* 7 (1995): 11–23.

L.D. Belkien, J. Bordt, O. Moller, et al., "Estradiol in Saliva for Monitoring Folliculae Stimulation in an In Vitro Fertilization Program," *Fertility and Sterility* 44 (3) (1985): 322–326.

F.L. Bellino, R.A. Saynes, P.J. Hornsby, et al., "Dehydroepiandrosterone (DHEA) and Aging," *The New York Academy of Sciences* (17–19 June 1995): 1–17.

Sarah L. Berga, "Transdermal HRT: New Trends, Emerging Targets," Contemporary OB/GYN Online CME course, September 2002.

Sarah L. Berga, "Sex Steroids and the Brain: Significance for Mental Health in Postmenopause," *Contemporary OB/GYN* (November 2001): 10–21.

S. Bhasin, T.W. Storer, N. Berman, et al., "The Effects of Supraphysiologic Doses of Testosterone on Muscle Size and Strength in Normal Men," *The New England Journal of Medicine* 335 (1) (1996): 1–4.

M.A. Birdsall, C.M. Farquhar, and H.D. White, "Association Between Polycystic Ovaries and Extent of Coronary Artery Disease in Women Having Cardiac Catheterization," *Annals of Internal Medicine* 126 (1) (1 January 1997): 32–35.

J.E. Buster, "Gestational Changes in Steroid Hormone Biosynthesis, Secretion, Metabolism, and Action," *Clinical Perinatology* 10 (1983): 527–552.

J.E. Buster, P.R. Casson, A.B. Straughn, et al., "Postmenopausal Steroid Replacement with Micronized Dehydroepiandrosterone: Preliminary Oral Bioavailability and Dose Proportionality Studies," *American Journal of Obstetrics and Gynecology* 166 (1992): 163–170.

B.C. Campbell and P.T. Ellison, "Menstrual Variations in Salivary Testosterone Among Regularly Cycling Women," *Hormone Research* 37 (1992): 132–136.

M.S. Canez, K.H. Lee, and D.L. Olive, "Progesterones and Estrogens," *Infertility and Reproduction Medical Clinics of North America* 3 (1992): 59–78.

R. Cannon, J. Ju Hsin-Shan, and C. Arnaud, "Analytical and Biological Variability of Three Bone Resorption Markers Affect Interpretation of Alendronate Response," *Bone* 20 (Supplement 4) (1997): 49S.

P.R. Casson, A.B. Straughn, E.S. Umstot, et al., "Delivery of Dehydroepiandrosterone to Premenopausal Women: Effects of Micronization and Non-oral Administration," *American Journal of Obstetrics and Gynecology* 174 (1996): 649–653.

A.H. Chakmakjian and N.Y. Zachariah, "Bioavailability of Progesterone with Different Modes of Administration," *The Journal of Reproductive Medicine* 32 (6) (1987): 443–447.

K.J. Chang, T.T.Y. Lee, G. Linares-Cruz, et al., "Influences of Percutaneous Administration of Estradiol and Progesterone on Human Breast Epithelial Cell Cycle in Vivo," *Chemistry* 43 (7) (1997): 1159–1164.

E. Cicinelli, D. deZiegler, P. Galantino, et al., "Twice-Weekly Transdermal Estradiol and Vaginal Progesterone as Continuous Combined Hormone Replacement Therapy in Postmenopausal Women: A 1-Year Prospective Study," *American Journal of Obstetrics and Gynecology* 187 (3) (September 2002): 556–560.

R.J. Cipolle, W.R. Crom, K. Crossley, et al., "Therapeutic Use and Serum Concentration Monitoring," in W.J. Taylor and A.L. Finn, eds., *Individualizing Drug Therapy: Practical Applications of Drug Monitoring* (New York: Gross, Townsend, Frank, Inc., 1981).

M.A. Cobleigh, R.F. Berris, T. Bush, et al., for the Breast Cancer Committees of the Eastern Cooperative Oncology Group, "Estrogen Replacement Therapy in Breast Cancer Survivors," *Journal of the American Medical Association* 272 (7) (1994): 540–545.

G.A. Colditz, S.E. Hankinson, D.J. Hunter, et al., "The Use of Estrogens and Progestins and the Risk of Breast Cancer in Post-menopausal Women," *The New England Journal of Medicine* 332 (15 June 1995): 1589–1593.

G.A..Colditz, M.J. Stampfer, W.C. Willett, et al., "Type of Postmenopausal Hormone Use and Risk of Breast Cancer: 12-year Follow-up from the Nurses' Health Study," *Cancer Causes and Control* 3 (1992): 433–439.

D.C. Cumming, M.E. Quigley, and S.S.C. Yen, "Acute Suppression of Circulating Testosterone Levels by Cortisol in Men," *Journal of Clinical Endocrinology and Metabolism* 57 (3) (1983): 671–673.

J. Dabbs, "Salivary Testosterone Measurements: Collecting, Storing, and Mailing Saliva Samples," *Physiology and Behavior* 49 (1991): 815–817.

J.M. Dabbs, "Salivary Testosterone Measurements in Behavioral Studies," *Annals of the New York Academy of Sciences* 49 (1991): 815–817.

J.M. Dabbs and S. Mohammed, "Male and Female Salivary Testosterone Concentrations Before and After Sexual Activity," *Physiology and Behavior* 52 (1992): 195–197.

R.H. Davies, B. Harris, D.R. Thomas, et al., "Salivary Testosterone Levels and Major Depressive Illness in Men," *British Journal of Psychiatry* 161 (1992): 629–632.

B. de Lignieres, "Effects of Progestogens on the Postmenopausal Breast," *Climacteric* 5 (3) (2002): 229–235.

B. de Lignieres, L. Dennerstein, and T. Backstrom, "Influence of Route of Administration on Progesterone Metabolism," *Maturitas* 21 (1995): 251–257.

M.J. De Souza, K.M. Prestwood, A.A. Luciano, et al., "A Comparison of the Effect of Synthetic and Micronized Hormone Replacement Therapy on Bone Mineral Density and Bio-chemical Markers of Bone Metabolism," *Menopause: The Journal of the North American Menopause Society* 3 (3) (1996): 140–148.

C. Dollbaum, J. Kells, H.M. Perry III, et al., "Validation of Salivary Testosterone as a Screening Test for Male Hypogonadism," abstract, Eighty-fifth Annual Meeting of The Endocrine Society, Charlottetown, Prince Edward Island, Canada, June 2003.

C.M. Dollbaum and G.S. Duwe, "Absorption of Progesterone After Topical Application: Serum and Saliva Level," presentation at the Seventh Annual Meeting of North American Menopause Society, San Francisco, CA, September 1995.

R.I. Dorfman and R.A. Shipley, *Androgens* (New York: John Wiley & Sons, 1959), 116–118.

A. Dupont, P. Dupont, L. Cusan, et al., "Comparative Endocrinological and Clinical Effects of Percutaneous Estradiol and Oral Conjugated Estrogens as Replacement Therapy in Menopausal Women," *Maturitas* 13 (1991): 297–311.

W.D. Dupont, D.L. Page, L.W. Rogers, et al., "Influence of Exogenous Estrogens, Proliferative Breast Disease, and Other Variables on Breast Cancer Risk," *Cancer* 63 (1989): 948–957.

P. Ebeling, L. Atley, J. Guthrie, et al., "Bone Turnover Markers and Bone Density Across the Menopausal Transition," *Journal of Clinical Endocrinology and Metabolism* 81 (9) (1996): 3366–3371.

J.A. Eden, "A Case-Control Study of Combined Continuous Estrogen-Progestin Replacement Therapy Among Women with a Personal History of Breast Cancer," *Menopause: The Journal of the North American Menopause Society* 2 (2) (1995): 67–72.

D.M. Eisenberg, R.C. Kessler, C. Foster, et al., "Unconventional Medicine in the United States, Prevalence, Costs and Patterns of Use," *The New England Journal of Medicine* 28 (Janaury 1993): 246–252.

P. Ellison, "Measurement of Salivary Progesterone," *Annals of the New York Academy of Sciences, 1992,* 161–176.

B. Ettinger, G.D. Friedman, T. Bush, et al., "Reducing Mortality Associated with Long-Term Postmenopausal Estrogen Therapy," *Obstetrics and Gynecology* 87 (1) (1996): 6–12.

A. Fisher and J.E. Morley, "Antiaging Medicine: The Good, the Bad and the Ugly," The *Journals of Gerontology. Series A, Biological Sciences and Medical Sciences* 57 (10) (October 2002): M636–M639.

I. Fogelman, "The Effects of Oestrogen Deficiency on the Skeleton and Its Prevention," *British Journal of Obstetrics and Gynecology* 14 (Supplement 103) (1996): 5–9.

A. Fulton, S. Chen, and G. Coleman, "Effect of Salivary Protein on Binding Curves of Three Radioimmunoassay Kits: Amerlex-M, Progesterone, Amerlex Cortisol, and Biodata Testosterone," *Clinical Chemistry* 35 (4) (1989): 641–644.

A.R. Gaby, "Dehydroepiandrosterone: Biological Effects and Clinical Significance," *Alternative Medicine Review* 1 (1996): 60–69.

R.D. Gambrell Jr., "Hormone Replacement Therapy in Patients with Previous Breast Cancer," *Menopause: The Journal of the North American Menopause Society* 2 (1995): 73–80.

P. Garnero, E. Hausherr, M.C. Chapuy, et al., "Markers of Bone Resorption Predict Hip Fracture in Elderly Women: The EPIDOS Prospective Study," *Journal of Bone and Mineral Research* 11 (1996): 1531–1538.

S.J. Gaskell, A.W. Pike, and K. Griffiths, "Analysis of Testosterone and Dehydroepiandrosterones in Saliva by Gas Chromatography-Mass Spectrometry," *Steroids* 36 (2) (1980): 218–229.

Margery L.S. Gass, Wulf Utian, Bruce Ettinger, et al., *Report from the NAMS Advisory Panel on Postmenopausal Hormone Therapy,* October 2002.

J.Y. Gillet, G. Andre, B. Faguer, et al., "Induction of Amenorrhea During Hormone Replacement Therapy: Optimal Micronized Progesterone Dose. A Multicenter Study," *Maturitas* 19 (1994): 103–115.

D. Grady, D. Herrington, V. Bittner, et al., for the HERS Research Group, "Cardiovascular Disease Outcomes During 6.8 Years of Hormone Therapy: Heart and Estrogen/Progestin Replacement Study Follow-up (HERS II)," *Journal of the American Medical Association* 288 (2002): 49–57.

D. Grady, S.M. Rubin, D.B. Petitti, et al., "Hormone Therapy to Prevent Disease and Prolong Life in Postmenopausal Women," *Annals of Internal Medicine* 117 (1992): 1016–1037.

R.A. Greene, "Estrogen and Cerebral Blood Flow: A Mechanism to Explain the Impact of Estrogen on the Incidence and Treatment of Alzheimer's Disease." *International Journal of Fertility and Women's Medicine* 45 (4) (July–August 2000): 253–257.

F. Grodstein, M.J. Stampfer, G.A. Colditz, et al., "Postmenopausal Hormone Therapy and Mortality," *The New England Journal of Medicine* 336 (1997): 1769–1775.

M.T. Haren, J.E. Morley, I.M. Chapman, et al., "Defining 'Relative' Androgen Deficiency in Aging Men: How Should Testosterone Be Measured, and What Are the Relationships Between Androgen Levels and Physical, Sexual and Emotional Health?" *Climacteric* 5 (1) (March 2002): 554–559.

J.T. Hargrove and E. Eisenberg, "Menopause," *Medical Clinics of North America* 79 (6) (1995): 1337–1356.

J.T. Hargrove, W. Maxson, and A.C. Wentz, "Absorption of Oral Progesterone Is Influenced by Vehicle and Particle Size," *American Journal of Obstetrics and Gynecology* 161 (1989): 948–951.

J.T. Hargrove, W.S. Maxson, A.C. Wentz, et al., "Menopausal Hormone Replacement Therapy with Continuous Daily Oral Micronized Estradiol and Progesterone," *Obstetrics and Gynecology* 73 (1989): 606–612.

J.T. Hargrove and K.G. Oseen, "An Alternative Method of Hormone Replacement Therapy Using the Natural Sex Steroids," *Menopause: The Journal of the North American Menopause Society* 6 (1995): 653–674.

L. Henriksson, M. Stjernquist, L. Boquist, et al., "A Comparative Multicenter Study of the Effects of Continuous Low-Dose Estradiol Released from a New Vaginal Ring Versus Estriol Vaginal Pessaries in Postmenopausal Women with Symptoms and Signs of Urogenital Atrophy," *American Journal of Obstetrics and Gynecology* 171 (1994): 624–632.

K. Howard, M. Kane, A. Madden, et al., "Direct Solid-Phase Enzymoimmunoassay of Testosterone in Saliva," *Clinical Chemistry* 35 (10) (1989): 2044–2047.

J.S. Hyams and D.E. Carey, "Corticosteroids and Growth," *Journal of Pediatrics* 1132 (1988): 249–254.

H. Jurz, H. Trunk, and B. Weitz, "Evaluation of Method to Determine Protein Binding of Drugs: Equilibrium Dialysis, Ultracentrifugation, Gel Filtration," *Drug Research* 27 (1977): 1373–1380.

A.M. Kanaya, D. Herrington, E. Vittinghoff, et al., "Glycemic Effects of Postmenopausal Hormone Therapy: The Heart and Estrogen/Progestin Replacement Study. A Randomized, Double-Blind, Placebo-Controlled Trial," *Annals of Internal Medicine* 138 (1) (7 January 2003): 1–9.

D.W. Kaufman, J.R. Palmer, J. De Mouzon, et al., "Estrogen Replacement Therapy and the Risk of Breast Cancer: Results from the Case-Control Surveillance Study," *American Journal of Epidemiology* 134 (1991): 1375–1385.

Patricia Kelly, "Recent HRT Studies: The Findings in Perspective," *San Francisco Medicine*, September 2002.

J.P. Keslak, "Can Estrogen Play a Significant Role in the Prevention of Alzheimer's Disease?" *Journal of Neural Transmission* (62) (Supplement) (2002): 227–239.

L.M. Kimzey, J. Fumowski, G. Merriman, et al., "Absorption of Micronized Progesterone from a Nonliquefying Vaginal Cream," *Fertility and Sterility* 56 (1991): 995–996.

C. Lauritzen, "Results of a Five-Year Prospective Study of Estriol Succinate Treatment in Patients with Climacteric Complaints," *Hormone Metabolism Research* 19 (1987): 579–584.

R. Leake, "Contents of HRT and Mechanisms of Action," *Journal of Epidemiology and Biostatistics* 4 (3) (1999): 129–133; discussion 133–139.

C.M. Lebrun, D.C. McKenzie, J.C. Prior, et al., "Effects of Menstrual Cycle Phase on Athletic Performance," *Medicine and Science in Sports and Exercise* 27 (3) (March 1995): 437–444.

I.M. Lee, R.S. Paffenbarger Jr., and C.H. Hennekens, "Physical Activity, Physical Fitness and Longevity," *Aging* (Milano) 9 (1–2) (February–April 1997): 2–11.

John R. Lee and Virginia Hopkins, *What Your Doctor May Not Tell You About Menopause: The Breakthrough Book on Natural Progesterone* (New York: Warner Books, 1996).

J.R. Lee, "Osteoporosis Reversal: The Role of Progesterone," *International Clinical Nutrition Review* 10 (3) (1990): 384–391.

H.M. Lemon, "Antimammary Carcinogenic Activity of 17-Alpha Ethinyl Estriol," *Cancer* 60 (12) (1987): 2873–2881.

H.M. Lemon, "Estriol, The Forgotten Estrogen?" *Journal of the American Medical Association* 239 (1) (1978): 29–30.

H.M. Lemon, H.H. Wotiz, L. Parsons, et al., "Reduced Estriol Excretion in Patients with Breast Cancer Prior to Endocrine Therapy," *Journal of the American Medical Association* 196 (13) (1966): 1128–1136.

H.B. Leonetti, K.J. Wilson, and J.N. Anasti, "Topical Progesterone Cream Has an Antiproliferative Effect on Estrogen-Stimulated Endometrium," *Fertility and Sterility* 79 (1) (January 2003): 221–222.

S. Lipson and P. Ellison, "Development of Protocols for the Application of Salivary Steroid Analysis to Field Conditions," *American Journal of Human Biology* 1 (1989): 249–255.

A.C. Looker, C.C. Johnson, H.W. Wahner, et al., "Prevalence of Low Femoral Bone Density in Older US Women from NHANES III," *Journal of Bone and Mineral Research* 10 (1995): 796–802.

L.J.W. Lu, K.E. Anderson, J.J. Grady, et al., "Effects of Soya Consumption for One Month on Steroid Hormones in Premenopausal Women: Implications for Breast Cancer Risk Reduction," *Cancer Epidemiology, Biomarkers, and Prevention* 5 (1) (January 1996): 63–70.

Y. Lu, R.T. Chatterton, K.M. Vogelsong, et al., "Direct Radioimmunoassay of Progesterone in Saliva," *Journal of Immunoassay* 18 (2) (1997): 149.

J.C. Marshall, "Hormonal Regulation of the Menstrual Cycle and Mechanisms of Anovulation," in Leslie Degroot, ed., *Endocrinology,* 3rd ed. (Philadelphia: W.B. Saunders Co., 1994), 2046–2057.

J. Martorano, M. Ahlgrimm, and T. Colbert, "Differentiating Between Natural Progesterone and Synthetic Progestins: Clinical Implications for Premenstrual Syndrome and Perimenopause Management," *Comprehensive Therapy* 24 (1998): 336–339.

T. Maruo, D.R. Mishell, A. Ben-Chetrit, et al., "Vaginal Rings Delivering Progesterone and Estradiol May Be a New Method of Hormone Replacement Therapy," *Fertility and Sterility* 78 (5) (November 2002): 1010–1016.

W.S. Maxson, "The Use of Progesterone in the Treatment of PMS," *Clinical Obstetrics and Gynecology* 30 (2) (1987): 465–468.

W.S. Maxson and J.T. Hargrove, "Bioavailability of Oral Micronized Progesterone," *Fertility and Sterility* 44 (1985): 622–626.

J.A. McGregor, G.M. Jackson, G.C.L. Lachelin, et al., "Salivary Estriol as Risk Assessment for Preterm Labor: A Prospective Trial," *American Journal of Obstetrics and Gynecology* 173 (1995): 1337–1342.

E.N. Meilahn, J.A. Cauley, R.P. Tracy, et al., "Association of Sex Hormones and Adiposity with Plasma Levels of Fibrinogen and PAI-1 in Postmenopausal Women," *American Journal of Epidemiology* 143 (2) (15 January 1996): 159–166.

G.B. Melis, A. Cagnacci, V. Bruni, et al., "Salmon Calcitonin Plus Intravaginal Estriol: An Effective Treatment for Menopause," *Maturitas* 24 (1–2) (1996): 83–90.

D. Michelson, C. Stratakis, L. Hill, et al., "Bone Mineral Density in Women with Depression," *The New England Journal of Medicine* 335 (1996): 1176–1181.

C.J. Migeon and R.L. Lanes, "Adrenal Cortex: Hypo- and Hyperfunction," in F. Lifshitz, ed., *Pediatric Endocrinology: A Clinical Guide,* 2d ed. (New York: Marcel Dekker, Inc., 1990), 333–352.

H. Minaguchi, T. Uemara, K. Shirasu, et al., "Effect of Estriol on Bone Loss in Postmenopausal Japanese Women: A Multicenter Prospective Open Study," *Journal of Obstetrics and Gynecology Research* 22 (3) (June 1996): 259–265.

D.R. Mishell and M.E. Mendelsohn, "Introduction: The Role of Hormone Replacement Therapy in Prevention and Treatment of Cardiovascular Disease in Postmenopausal Women," *American Journal of Cardiology* 89 (Supplement 12) (2002): 1E–4E.

P.E. Mohr, D.Y. Wang, W.M. Gregory, et al., "Serum Progesterone and Prognosis in Operable Breast Cancer," *British Journal of Cancer* 73 (1996): 1552–1555.

S.E. Monroe and K.M.J. Menon, "Changes in Reproductive Hormone Secretion During the Climacteric and Postmenopausal Periods," *Clinical Obstetrics and Gynecology* 20 (1977): 113–122.

A.J. Morales, J.J. Nolan, J.C. Nelson, et al., "Effects of Replacement Dose of Dehydroepiandrosterone in Men and Women of Advancing Age," *Journal of Clinical Endocrinology and Metabolism* 781 (1994): 1360–1367.

J.E. Morley, P. Patrick, and M.N. Perry III, "Evaluation of Assays Available to Measure Free Testosterone," *Metabolism* 51 (5) (May 2002): 554–559.

D.L. Moyer, B. de Lignieres, P. Driguez, et al., "Prevention of Endometrial Hyperplasia by Progesterone During Long-Term Estradiol Replacement: Influence of Bleeding Pattern and Secretory Changes," *Fertility and Sterility* 59 (1993): 992–997.

A. Munck, P. Guyre, N. Holbrook, et al., "Physiological Actions of Glucocorticoids in Stress and Their Relation to Pharmacological Actions," *Endocrine Review* 5 (1984): 25.

H.D. Nelson, L.L. Humphrey, P. Nygren, et al., "Postmenopausal Hormone Replacement Therapy: Scientific Review," *Journal of the American Medical Association (JAMA)* 288 (2002): 872–881.

A. Nishibe, S. Morimoto, K. Hirota, et al., "Effect of Estriol and Bone Mineral Density of Lumbar Vertebrae in Elderly and Postmenopausal Women," *Nippon Romen Igakkai Zasshi* [Japanese Journal of Geriatrics] 33 (5) (1996): 353–359.

T.R. Norman, C.A. Morse, and L. Dennerstein, "Comparative Bioavailability of Orally and Vaginally Administered Progesterone," *Fertility and Sterility* 56 (1991): 1034–1039.

Morris Notelovitz, "Why Individualizing Hormone Therapy Is Crucial: Putting the Results of the WHI Trial into Perspective," *Medscape Women's Health eJournal* 7(4) (2002).

M. Nozaki, K. Hashimoto, Y. Inoue, et al., "Usefulness of Estriol for the Treatment of Bone Loss in Postmenopausal Women," *Nippon Sanka Fujinka Gakkai Zasshi* [Japanese Journal of Obstetrics and Gynecology] 48 (2) (February 1996): 83–88.

W.D. Odell, "The Menopause and Hormonal Replacement," in Leslie Degroot, ed., *Endocrinology,* 3rd ed. (Philadelphia: W.B. Saunders Co., 1994), 2128–2139.

T. Ojasoo, J.P. Raynaud, and J.C. Dore, "Affiliations Among Steroid Receptors as Revealed by Multivariate Analysis of Steroid Binding Data," *Journal of Steroid Biochemistry and Molecular Biology* 48 (1994): 31–46.

D.A. Oriba, D. Bucks, and H. Maibach, "Percutaneous Absorption of Hydrocortisone and Testosterone on the Vulva and Forearm: Effect of the Menopause and Site," *British Journal of Dermatology* 134 (1996): 229–233.

A. O'Rorke, M.M. Kane, J.P. Gosling, et al., "Development and Validation of a Monoclonal Antibody Enzyme Immunoassay for Measuring Progesterone in Saliva," *Clinical Chemistry* 403 (1994): 454–458.

M.L. Padwick, N.C. Siddle, G. Lane, et al., "Oestriol with Oestradiol Versus Oestradiol Alone: A Comparison of Endometrial, Symptomatic and Psychological Effects," *British Journal of Obstetrics and Gynecology* 93 (June 1986): 606–612.

A. Paganini-Hill and V.W. Henderson, "Estrogen Replacement Therapy and Risk of Alzheimer's Disease," *Archives of Internal Medicine* 156 (1996): 2213–2217.

J.R. Palmer, L. Rosenberg, E.A. Clarke, et al., "Breast Cancer Risk After Estrogen Replacement Therapy: Results from the Toronto Breast Cancer Study," *American Journal of Epidemiology* 134 (1991): 1386–1395.

N. Panay and J. Studd, "Do Progestogens and Progesterone Reduce Bone Loss?" *Menopause: Journal of the North American Menopause Society* 3 (1) (1996): 13–19.

F.R. Perez-Lopez, C. Campo-Lopez, L. Alos, et al., "Oestrogen and Progesterone Receptors in the Human Vagina During the Menstrual Cycle, Pregnancy and Postmenopause," *Maturitas* 16 (1993): 139–144.

T. Perls, L. Alpert, and R. Fretts, "Middle-Aged Mothers Live Longer," *Nature* 389 (1997): 133.

N.L. Petrakis, S. Barnes, E.B. King, et al., "Stimulatory Influence of Soy Protein Isolate on Breast Secretion in Pre- and Postmenopausal Women," *Cancer Epidemiology, Biomarkers, and Prevention* 5 (10) (1996): 785–794.

G.B. Phillips, B.H. Pindernell, and T.Y. Jing, "Relationship Between Serum Sex Hormones and Coronary Artery Disease in Postmenopausal Women," *Arteriosclerosis and Thrombosis in Vascular Biology* 17 (4) (April 1997): 695–701.

C. Picado and M. Luengo, "Corticosteroid-Induced Bone Loss: Prevention and Management," *Drug Safety* 15 (5) (November 1996): 347–359.

M. Powers, L. Schenkel, P.E. Darley, et al., "Pharmacokinetics and Pharmacodynamics of Transdermal Dosage Forms of 17 B-Estradiol: Comparison with Conventional Oral Estrogens Used for Hormone Replacement," *American Journal of Obstetrics and Gynecology* 152 (1985): 1099–1106.

J.H. Price, H. Ismail, R.H. Gorwill, et al., "Effect of the Suppository Base on Progesterone Delivery from the Vagina," *Fertility and Sterility* 39 (1983): 490–493.

J.C. Prior, "Progesterone and the Prevention of Osteroporosis," *Canadian Journal of Ob/Gyn and Women's Health Care* 3 (1991): 13–19.

J.C. Prior, "Progesterone as a Bone-Trophic Hormone," *Endocrine Review* 11 (May 1990): 386–398.

J.C. Prior, Y.M. Vigna, and D.W. McKay, "Reproduction for the Athletic Woman: New Understandings of Physiology and Management," *Sports Medicine* 14 (3) (1992): 190–199.

J. Prior, Y.M. Vigna, M.T. Schechter, et al., "Spinal Bone Loss and Ovulatory Disturbances," *The New England Journal of Medicine* 323 (1 November 1990): 1221–1227.

J.G. Rabkin, R. Rabkin, and G. Wagner, "Testosterone Replacement Therapy in HIV Illness," *General Hospital Psychiatry* 17 (1) (January 1955): 37–42.

N.F. Ray, J.K. Chan, M. Thamer, et al., "Medical Expenditures for the Treatment of Osteoporotic Fractures in the United States in 1995: Report from the National Osteoporosis Foundation," *Journal of Bone and Mineral Research* 12 (1997): 24–35.

R. Raz and W.E. Stamm, "A Controlled Trial of Intravaginal Estriol in Postmenopausal Women with Recurrent Urinary Tract Infections," *The New England Journal of Medicine* 329 (1993): 753–756.

G.F. Read, "Status Report on Measurement of Salivary Estrogens and Androgens," *Annals of the New York Academy of Sciences, 1993,* 146–160.

W. Regelson, R. Lovia, and M. Kalimi, "Dehydroepiandrosterone (DHEA) the 'Mother Steroid,' " *Annals of the New York Academy of Sciences* 719 (1994): 552–563.

W. Regelson, R. Lovia, and M. Kalimi, "Hormonal Intervention: 'Buffer Hormones' or 'State Dependency.' The Role of Dehydroepiandrosterone (DHEA), Thyroid Hormone, Estrogen and Hypophysectomy in Aging," *Annals of the New York Academy of Sciences* 521 (1988): 260–273.

R. Reid, "Pathogenesis and Treatment of Steroid Osteoporosis," *Clinical Endocrinology* 30 (1989): 83–103.

D. Riad-Fahmy, G.F. Read, and R.F. Walker, "Salivary Steroid Assays for Assessing Variation in Endocrine Activity," *Journal of Steroid Biochemistry* 19 (1983): 265–272.

V. Montgomery Rice, "Hormone Replacement Therapy: Optimizing the Dose and Route of Administration," *Drugs and Aging* 19 (11) (2002): 807–818.

B.L. Riggs, "Overview of Osteoporosis," *Western Journal of Medicine* 154 (January 1991): 63–77.

J. Robel, J. Young, C. Corpechot, et al., "Biosynthesis and Assay of Neurosteroids in Rats and Mice; Functional Correlates," *Journal of Steroid Biochemistry and Molecular Biology* 53 (1995): 355.

S.P. Robins, "Collagen Crosslinks in Metabolic Bone Disease," *Acta Orthopaedica Scandinavica* 66 (Supplement 266) (1995): 171–175.

S.P. Robins, H. Woitge, R. Hesley, et al., "Direct Enzyme-Linked Immunoassay for Urinary Deoxypyridinoline as a Specific Marker for Measuring Bone Resorption," *Journal of Bone and Mineral Research* 9 (1994): 1643–1649.

T.E. Rohan and A.J. McMichael, "Non-contraceptive Exogenous Oestrogen Therapy and Breast Cancer," *Medical Journal of Australia* 148 (1988): 217–221.

T.H. Sannikka, P. Terho, J. Suominen, et al., "Testosterone Concentration in Human Seminal Plasma and Saliva and Its Correlations with Non Protein-Bound and Total Testosterone Levels in Serum," *International Journal of Andrology* 6 (1983): 319–330.

L. Schenkel, D. Barlier, M. Riera, et al., "Transdermal Absorption of Estradiol from Different Body Sites Is Comparable," *Journal of Controlled Release* 4 (1986): 195–201.

R. Schlaghecke, E. Komely, R.T. Santen, et al., "The Effect of Long-Term Glucocorticoid on Pituitary-Adrenal Responses to Exogenous Corticotropin-Releasing Hormone," *The New England Journal of Medicine* 326 (1992): 226–230.

R.T. Scott Jr., B. Ross, C. Anderson, et al., "Pharmacokinetics of Percutaneous Estradiol: A Crossover Study Using a Gel and a Transdermal System in Comparison with Oral Micronized Estradiol," *Obstetrics and Gynecology* 77 (1991): 758–764.

P.M. Serrel, "How Progestins Compromise the Cardioprotective Effects of Estrogens," *Menopause* 2 (1995): 187–190.

E. Shane, M. Rivas, D.J. McMahon, et al., "Bone Loss and Turnover After Cardiac Transplantation," *Journal of Clinical Endocrinology and Metabolism* 82 (5) (May 1997): 1497–1506.

C.N. Shealy, "A Review of Dehydroepiandrosterone (DHEA)," *Integrative Physiological and Behavioral Science* 30 (4) (September–December 1995): 308–313.

B.B. Sherwin, "The Impact of Different Doses of Estrogen and Progestin on Mood and Sexual Behavior in Postmenopause," *Journal of Clinical Endocrinology and Metabolism* 72 (1991): 336–343.

M. Shimada, K. Takahashi, T. Ohkawa, et al., "Determination of Salivary Cortisol by ELISA and Its Application into the Assessment of the Circadian Rhythm in Children," *Hormone Research* 44 (1995): 213.

J.W. Simkins, P.S. Green, K.E. Gridley, et al., "Role of Estrogen Replacement Therapy in Memory Enhancement and the Prevention of Neuronal Loss Associated with Alzheimer's Disease," *American Journal of Medicine* 103 (1997): 19s–25s.

J.A. Simon, D.E. Robinson, M.C. Andrews, et al., "The Absorption of Oral Micronized Progesterone: The Effect of Food, Dose Proportionality, and Comparison with Intramuscular Progesterone," *Fertility and Sterility* 60 (1993): 26–33.

R. Sodergard, T. Backstrom, V. Shanbhag, et al., "Calculation of Free and Bound Fractions of Testosterone and Estradiol-17B to Human Plasma Proteins at Body Temperature," *Journal of Steroid Biochemistry* 16 (1982): 801–810.

Leon Speroff, "Response to the WHI by Clinicians," *OB/GYN Clinical Alert,* December 2002: 57–59.

Leon Speroff, "Hormone Replacement Therapy: Clarifying the Picture," *Hospital Practice* 36 (5) (May 2001): 44–45; discussion 45–46.

L. Speroff, R.H. Glass, and N.G. Kase, *Clinical Gynecologic Endocrinology and Infertility,* 3rd ed. (Baltimore: Williams & Wilkins, 1983).

J.L. Stanford, N.S. Weiss, L.F. Voigt, et al., "Combined Estrogen and Progestin Hormone Replacement Therapy in Relation to Risk of Breast Cancer in Middle-Aged Women," *Journal of the American Medical Association* 274 (1995): 137–142.

P.M. Stewart, J.R. Secl, J. Corrie, et al., "A Rational Approach for Assessing the Hypothalamo-Pituitary-Adrenal Axis," *Lancet* 5 (1988): 1208–1210.

J. Studd, "Current Option: Hormone Replacement Therapy After a Diagnosis of Breast Cancer," *Menopause: The Journal of the North American Menopause Society* 2 (1995): 55–57.

B. Sufi, A. Donaldson, S.C. Gandy, et al., "Multicenter Evaluation of Assays for Estradiol and Progesterone in Saliva," *Clinical Chemistry* 31 (1) (1985): 101–103.

E. Talbott, D. Guzick, A. Clerici, et al., "Coronary Heart Disease Risk Factors in Women with Polycystic Ovary Syndrome," *Arteriosclerosis and Thrombosis in Vascular Biology* 15 (7) (July 1995): 821–826.

K. Tamate, M. Charleton, J.P. Gosling, et al., "Direct Colorimetric Monoclonal Antibody Enzyme Immunoassay for Estradiol 17-B in Saliva," *Clinical Chemistry* 43 (1997): 1159–1164.

K.H. Tennekoon and E.H. Karunanayake, "Serum FSH, LH, and Testosterone Concentrations in Fertile Men: Effect of Age," *International Journal of Fertility* 38 (2) (1993): 108–112.

H.L. Thacker, "The Case for Hormone Replacement: New Studies That Should Inform the Debate," *Cleveland Clinic Journal of Medicine* 69 (9) (September 2002): 670–678.

H. Tobe, O. Komiyama, Y. Komiyama, et al., "Stimulation of Bone Resorption in Pit Formation Assay," *Bioscience, Biotechnology, and Biochemistry* 61 (2) (1997): 370–371.

T. Tomita, F. Sawamura, R. Uetsuka, et al., "Inhibition of Cholesterylester Accumulation by 17beta Estradiol in Macrophages Through Activation of Neutral Cholesterol Esterase," *Biochimica et Biophysica Acta* 1300 (3) (20 May 1996): 210–218.

P.G. Toniolo, M. Levitz, A. Zeleniuch-Jacquotte, et al., "A Prospective Study of Endogenous Estrogens in Breast Cancer in Postmenopausal Women," *Journal of the National Cancer Institute* 87 (1995): 190–197.

S. Tunn, H. Mollmann, J. Barht, et al., "Simultaneous Measurement of Cortisol in Serum and Saliva After Different Forms of Cortisol Administration," *Clinical Chemistry* 38 (1992): 1491–1494.

Wulf Utian, "Managing Menopause After HERS II and WHI: Coping with the Aftermath," *Menopause Management* (July–August 2002): 6–7.

P.L. VanDaele, "Case Control Analysis of Bone Resorption Markers, Disability and Hip Fracture Risk: The Rotterdam Study," *British Medical Journal* 312 (7029) (24 February 1996): 482–483.

W. Vanselow, L. Dennerstein, K.M. Greenwood, et al., "Effects of Progesterone and Its 5A and 5B Metabolites on Symptoms of Premenstrual Syndrome According to Route of Administration," *Journal of Psychosomatic Obstetrics and Gynecology* 17 (1996): 29–38.

J.C. Vera, A.M. Reyes, J.G. Carcamo, et al., "Genistein Is a Natural Inhibitor of Dehydroascorbic Acid Transport Through the Glucose Transporter, GLUT1," *Journal of Biological Chemistry* 271 (1996): 8719–8724.

A. Vermeulen and J.M. Kaufman, "Aging of the Hypothalamo-Pituitary-Testicular Axis in Men," *Hormone Research* 43 (1995): 25–28.

R.F. Vining and R.A. McGinley, "The Measurement of Hormones in Saliva: Possibilities and Pitfalls," *Journal of Steroid Biochemistry* 27 (1987): 81–94.

R.F. Vining, R.A. McGinley, and R.G. Symons, "Hormones in Saliva: Mode of Entry and Consequent Implications for Clinical Interpretation," *Clinical Chemistry* 29 (10) (1983): 1752–1756.

J. Vitteck, G.D. L'Hommedieu, F.F. Fordon, et al., "Direct Radio-Immunoassay RIA of Salivary Testosterone Correlation with Free and Total Serum Testosterone," *Life Sciences* 37 (1985): 711–716.

O.J. Vrieze, J. Kuipers, and G.J. Boes, "Scenario Analysis in Public Health and Competing Risks," *Statistics Applications* 1 (1990): 371–377.

S.E. Wade, "An Oral-Diffusion-Sink Device for Extended Sampling of Multiple Steroid Hormones from Saliva," *Clinical Chemistry* 38 (1992): 1878–1882.

C. Wang, S. Plymate, E. Nieschlag, et al., "Salivary Testosterone in Men: Further Evidence of a Direct Correlation with Free Serum Testosterone," *Journal of Clinical Endocrinology and Metabolism* 53 (1981): 1021.

M.J. Wheeler, "The Determination of Bio-available Testosterone," *Annals of Clinical Biochemistry* 82 (1995): 345.

U.H. Winkler, "Effects of Androgens on Haemostasis," *Maturitas* 24 (3) (July 1996): 147–155.

A.J. Wood, ed., "Drug Therapy Androgens in Men—Uses and Abuses," *The New England Journal of Medicine* 14 (March 1996): 707–714.

C.M. Worthman, J.F. Stallings, and L. Hofman, "Sensitive Salivary Estradiol Assay for Monitoring Ovarian Function," *Clinical Chemistry* 36 (1990): 1769–1773.

Writing Group for the PEPI Trial, "The Postmenopausal Estrogen/Progestin Interventions (PEPI) Trial: Effects of Estrogen or Estrogen/Progestin Regimens on Heart Disease Risk Factors in Postmenopausal Women," *Journal of the American Medical Association* 273 (1996): 199–208.

Writing Group for the PEPI Trial, "The Postmenopausal Estrogen/Progestin Interventions (PEPI) Trial: Effects of Hormone Replacement on Endometrial Histology in Postmenopausal Women," *Journal of the American Medical Association* 275 (1996): 370–375.

C.P. Yang, J.R. Daling, P.R. Band, et al., "Noncontraceptive Hormone Use and Risk of Breast Cancer," *Cancer Causes and Control* 3 (1992): 475–479.

T.S. Yang, S.H. Tsan, S.P. Chang, et al., "Efficacy and Safety of Estriol Replacement Therapy for Climacteric Women," *American Journal of Obstetrics and Gynecology* 173 (1995): 670–671.

S. Yen, A.J. Morales, and O. Khorram, "Replacement of DHEA in Aging Men and Women: Potential Remedial Effects," *Annals of the New York Academy of Sciences* 774 (1995): 128–142.

D.T. Zava, M. Blen, and G. Duwe, "Estrogenic Activity of Natural and Synthetic Estrogens in Human Breast Cancer Cells in Culture," *Environmental Health Perspectives* 105 (Supplement 3) (1997): 637–645.

D.T. Zava and G. Duwe, "Estrogenic and Antiproliferative Properties of Genistein and Other Flavonoids in Human Breast Cancer Cells in Vitro," *Nutrition and Cancer* 27 (1) (1997): 31–40.

B. Zunoff, G.W. Strain, L.K. Miller, et al., "24-Hour Mean Plasma Testosterone Concentration Declines with Age in Normal Premenopausal Women," *Journal of Clinical Endocrinology and Metabolism* 80 (4) (April 1995): 1429–1430.

GLOSSARY

adrenal glands Two small glands near the tops of the kidneys that produce glucocorticoids, mineralocorticoids, androgenic hormones, and the stress hormones epinephrine and norepinephrine.

adrenaline *See* Epinephrine.

amenorrhea Absence of menstruation.

anabolic General term for substances that stimulate growth.

anabolic hormone Any hormone that stimulates bone and muscle growth.

androgen A class of hormones produced by the adrenal glands in both sexes and in the ovaries in women and the testes in men. Testosterone, DHEA, and androstenedione are androgens. Women produce androgens in smaller amounts than men; however, levels decline with age in persons of both sexes.

androgenic A term used to describe natural or synthetic substances that can produce masculine characteristics, including male pattern hair growth, oily skin, acne, a deeper voice, increased appetite, and increased muscle mass.

androstenedione A sex steroid hormone that is secreted by the testis, ovary, and adrenal cortex, and acts in the production of masculine characteristics.

animal-derived Substances that come from animal source material. Equilin, the form of estrogen that comes from the urine of pregnant mares, is an example.

antibodies   Proteins that act specifically against an antigen in an immune response. Also referred to as *immunoglobulin*.

antigen   Any substance that stimulates an immune response.

antioxidant   A substance that combats free radicals in the body. Examples include beta-carotene, vitamins C and E, and the mineral selenium.

baseline   Data used for comparison or as a control.

bioavailable hormone   An active, or free, hormone that can bind with a receptor and create a response in tissue.

bisphosphonates   Drugs used in the prevention and treatment of osteoporosis. They work by being incorporated into the bone in an attempt to protect it from osteoclasts, the cells that break down bone.

bone resorption   The loss or breakdown of bone cells.

bound hormone   A hormone that is bound to sex hormone binding globulin (SHBG). These hormones are part of total blood-hormone levels but are not active in the body.

breakthrough bleeding   Irregular or prolonged uterine bleeding due to continual sloughing of the endometrium that is sometimes related to the use of HRT or oral contraceptives.

calcitonin   A hormone secreted by the thyroid gland that lowers the level of calcium in the blood. Also called *thyrocalcitonin*.

cardiovascular disease (CVD)   General term for diseases involving the heart, veins, arteries, and capillaries.

cascade effect   A series of sequential molecular or biochemical interactions that result in a physiologic change. The hormone cascade, which is the conversion of one sex steroid hormone into another (with the assistance of enzymes), is one example.

cell   The smallest structural unit of living matter capable of performing all the fundamental functions of life, either by itself or by interacting with other cells.

cholesterol   A steroid component of animal fats that regulates membrane fluidity, functions as a precursor molecule in the formation of sex steroid hormones, and is a constituent of both HDL (which protects against plaque formation in the arteries) and LDL (which can cause it). It is produced by the liver or obtained in certain foods.

circadian rhythm   Fluctuations in biological activity or function occurring in approximately twenty-four-hour cycles.

clotting factors   Plasma components such as fibrinogen that are involved in blood clotting.

compounding pharmacy   A pharmacy that specializes in formulating and making prescriptions by hand to suit individual patient needs.

conjugate   A chemical formed by the union of one compound with another.

conjugated estrogens   Term used to refer to a mixture of estrogens commonly used for hormone replacement in women. An example is Premarin, which is a combination of horse estrogens.

corticosteroid   Any steroid produced by the adrenal cortex. Examples include cortisol, DHEA, and pregnenolone.

cortisol   A glucocorticoid produced by the adrenal cortex commonly known as the stress hormone. It is a derivative of cortisone and helps the body cope with stresses of all kinds.

cortisone   A glucocorticoid produced both naturally by the adrenal glands and also synthetically that has powerful anti-inflammatory effects. As a drug, it is used to treat many different diseases and conditions.

creatinine   A type of protein found in muscle, blood, and urine.

dehydroepiandrosterone (DHEA)   A sex steroid hormone produced in the adrenal glands, the skin, and the brain. DHEA is associated with levels of vigor and vitality and the rate of aging.

delivery system   The way in which a drug is delivered into the body. Examples include oral tablets and capsules, which are taken by mouth; transdermal forms, which are absorbed through the skin; and sublingual forms, which are placed under the tongue and absorbed through the mucous membranes of the mouth.

deoxypyridinoline (Dpd)   A by-product of the breakdown of a type of collagen that exists in bone. Measuring the Dpd that is excreted unmetabolized in urine is a way of determining your rate of bone resorption (loss).

dihydrotestosterone (DHT)   DHT is a potent androgen that has been associated with hair loss in men and women. DHT is metabolized from testosterone by the enzyme conversion of 5-alpha reductase.

diosgenin   A chemical derived from the wild-yam plant that is used to make natural, identical-to-human hormones such as estradiol and progesterone. This conversion must be done in a laboratory, because the human body is unable to convert this compound into sex steroid hormones.

diurnal variation   A cycle or rhythm of activity that varies over the course of a day.

dopamine   A neurotransmitter in the brain that is important in the production of epinephrine (adrenaline).

down-regulating   Decreasing the number of active hormone receptors.

drug half-life   The time it takes to reduce a drug's blood concentration by half as a result of metabolism and excretion.

endocrine gland   A gland that produces hormones. Also called a *ductless gland* or *gland of internal secretion.*

endocrine system   The system of glands that produces endocrine secretions and helps regulate and control bodily metabolic activity. Includes the pituitary, thyroid, parathyroid, and adrenal glands as well as the pancreas, ovaries, and testes.

endometrial hyperplasia   An abnormal or unusual increase in the cellular layers of the endometrium.

endometrium   The mucous membrane lining the uterus.

enterohepatic recirculation   A situation in which a substance or molecule, like a hormone, passes through the gastrointestinal tract and reenters your system instead of being eliminated from the body.

enzymes   Complex proteins produced by living cells that assist in specific biochemical reactions in the body.

epinephrine   A hormone secreted by the adrenal glands whose effects are the classic fight-or-flight response. It increases heart function and raises blood-sugar levels. Epinephrine can also be prepared from adrenal extracts or made synthetically. In this form, it is used medicinally as a heart stimulant and as a vasoconstrictor to control hemorrhages of the skin. It is also used to prolong the effects of local anesthetics, as a muscle relaxant for bronchial asthma, and to counteract life-threatening allergic reactions. Also known as *adrenaline.*

equilin   An estrogenic steroid hormone occurring in the urine of pregnant mares and commonly used in human estrogen replacement therapy.

estradiol   The primary and most potent estrogenic hormone present in humans.

estriol   A naturally occurring but relatively weak human estrogen present in large amounts in pregnant women.

estrogen   A category of sex hormones produced by the ovary that includes estradiol, estrone, and estriol. Estrogens stimulate the development of female secondary sex characteristics.

estrone   An estrogenic hormone found circulating in higher amounts after menopause.

ethinyl estradiol   A potent synthetic oral estrogen used mainly for birth control.

feedback   The process by which the products of a cascade affect their own production either negatively or positively.

fibrocystic breasts   Breasts that have developed lumpy fibrous tissue and cysts.

fibroid   *See* Uterine fibroid.

first-pass elimination   The breaking down, inactivation, and/or elimination of hormones from the bloodstream when they pass through the liver, directly after absorption from the gut.

follicle-stimulating hormone (FSH)   A hormone produced by the pituitary gland that stimulates the growth of the egg-containing follicles in the ovary and that activates sperm-forming cells in the testes.

follicular phase   The first half of the menstrual cycle that leads to ovulation. Estrogen dominates this part of the cycle.

fracture   Medical term for a broken bone.

free hormone   An active or bioavailable hormone circulating in the bloodstream.

free radical A highly reactive atom or group of atoms that can easily bind with other compounds and attack and damage cells and/or DNA.

gamma-aminobutyric acid (GABA) An amino acid that is a neurotransmitter in the central nervous system. It has a calming effect.

genistein A plant-derived hormone found in soybeans that has a molecular structure very similar to that of human estrogen and that may have estrogenic effects.

gland An organ or group of cells that selectively removes materials from the blood, concentrates or alters them, and secretes them for further use in the body or for elimination.

glucocorticoid A type of corticosteroid involved in carbohydrate, protein, and fat metabolism. They tend to increase liver-glycogen and blood-sugar levels and can reduce inflammation and suppress the immune response. Examples include hydrocortisone and dexamethasone. In medicine, glucocorticoids are used to alleviate symptoms of various conditions, including rheumatoid arthritis and asthma.

HDL A blood protein that carries cholesterol to the liver for excretion. It is known as "good cholesterol" because it is associated with a decreased probability of plaque formation and development of atherosclerosis. HDL stands for *high-density lipoprotein*.

hirsutism Excessive growth of hair on face or body.

hormonal diurnal variation Normal variation in hormone levels at different times of the day. For example, cortisol and testosterone levels are normally higher in the morning and lower at night. Melatonin levels are normally higher in the middle of the night and lower in the morning.

hormone Any one of a group of molecules produced by the endocrine glands that circulate throughout the bloodstream as chemical messengers and regulate many bodily functions.

hormone receptor A chemical structure that binds with a specific hormone and signals a cell for change.

hormone replacement therapy (HRT) The administration of hormones to make up for the loss of the body's own hormones that occurs with aging.

hot flash A menopausal symptom resulting from diminishing hormone levels that creates a physical sensation of a rapid change in temperature, from cool and clammy to hot and sweaty.

hyperplasia An abnormal or unusual increase in the number of cells composing a tissue.

hyperthyroidism A condition characterized by an overly active thyroid gland. Symptoms range from racing or jumpy heartbeat to anxiety, frequent loose stools, insomnia, and weight loss.

hypothalamus A gland at the base of the brain that regulates and controls the endocrine glands through its release of hormones. These hormones travel to the pituitary gland and in turn stimulate the release of pituitary hormones.

hypothyroidism A condition characterized by an underactive thyroid gland. Symptoms include a lowered metabolic rate and general loss of vigor, as well as loss of appetite, inability to tolerate cold, weight gain, muscle weakness and cramps, hair loss, dry skin, constipation, and depression.

hysterectomy   Surgical removal of the uterus.

immune system   The bodily system that protects the body from foreign substances, cells, and tissues by producing the immune response. Its components include the thymus; spleen; lymph nodes; special deposits of lymphoid tissue, such as those found in the gastrointestinal tract and bone marrow; specialized white blood cells known as lymphocytes, which include the B-cells and T-cells; and antibodies.

insomnia   Prolonged and abnormal inability to obtain adequate sleep.

insulin   A hormone secreted by the pancreas that is essential for the metabolism of carbohydrates. Medically, it is used in the treatment and control of diabetes.

isoflavone   A class of phytoestrogens (plant estrogens) that are found almost exclusively in legumes such as soybeans and include the compounds genistein and daidzein.

LDL   A blood protein that carries cholesterol throughout the bloodstream. It is known as "bad cholesterol" because it is associated with an increased probability of plaque formation and development of atherosclerosis. LDL stands for *low-density lipoprotein*.

libido   The emotional or psychic energy that is sexual drive, desire, and energy. It is associated with the sex steroid hormone testosterone.

long-chain fatty acid   A type of organic acid found predominantly in oils.

luteal phase   The second half of the menstrual cycle, from ovulation until menstruation begins. Progesterone dominates this part of the cycle.

luteinizing hormone (LH)   A hormone secreted by the pituitary gland that induces ovulation and the production of estradiol and progesterone, hormones associated with the menstrual cycle. In men, LH stimulates the testes to produce testosterone.

medroxyprogesterone acetate   A synthetic progesterone used to treat hormonal imbalance. An example is Provera.

melatonin   A hormone secreted by the pineal gland in response to darkness. It has been linked to the regulation of sleep.

menopause   The period of natural cessation of menstruation occurring usually between the ages of forty-five and fifty-two. At this time, the production of estradiol and progesterone diminishes, resulting in the cessation of ovulation and endometrial changes. Also called *the climacteric*.

menstrual cycle   The whole cycle of hormonal and physiologic changes from the beginning of one menstrual period to the beginning of the next.

menstruation   The discharge of blood, secretions, and tissue debris from the uterus that recurs every month in women, from puberty to menopause, when they do not become pregnant after ovulation.

metabolism   The process by which energy is produced and substances are created by living cells for the vital activities of the body.

metabolite A substance created by metabolism. A metabolite can be something that is essential to the organism or the metabolic process, or it can be a waste product that is toxic and meant to be excreted.

microgram One-millionth of a gram.

micronize To reduce the size of a particle to only a few microns (a micron equals one-millionth of a meter).

milligram One-thousandth of a gram.

milliliter One-thousandth of a liter.

mineralocorticoids Corticosteroids such as aldosterone that chiefly affect the electrolyte and fluid balance in the body.

molecule The smallest particle of a substance that retains all the properties of the substance. Molecules are composed of one or more atoms.

myelin sheath A protective covering around nerve fibers.

nanogram One-billionth of a gram.

natural hormones Replacement hormones that are synthesized from plant compounds derived from soy and wild yams. Natural replacement hormones are identical to human hormones.

natural hormone replacement therapy (NHRT) The use of natural, identical-to-human hormones to restore declining hormone levels.

natural killer cells Immune cells that kill tumor cells.

neuron A cell that transmits and receives nervous impulses; a nerve cell.

neurotransmitter A substance that transmits nerve impulses from one nerve cell to another. Examples include norepinephrine, acetylcholine, GABA, and serotonin.

norephinephrine (noradrenaline) A hormone secreted by the adrenal glands in response to hypertension and physical stress. It has a calming effect, the opposite of adrenaline.

nucleus The central portion of the cell that contains the genetic material (DNA). The nucleus is essential in governing cell functions such as reproduction and protein synthesis.

oophorectomy Surgical removal of the ovaries.

osteoblast A bone-building cell.

osteoclast A cell that breaks down bone.

osteopenia A reduction in bone density due to inadequate replacement of bone that has been lost. It can be a step on the path to osteoporosis.

osteoporosis A disease characterized by a decrease in bone mass, with decreased bone density and increased porosity and fragility.

ovary An essential female reproductive organ that produces eggs and sex steroid hormones.

ovulation The release of a mature ovum (egg) from the ovary. It occurs approximately halfway through the menstrual cycle.

pancreas   A gland that secretes digestive enzymes and the hormones insulin and glucagon.

parathyroid   Any of four small endocrine glands that are adjacent to or embedded in the thyroid gland. These glands produce parathyroid hormone, which regulates the metabolism of calcium and phosphorus in the body.

peak level   The highest concentration in blood or saliva that is achieved following ingestion or application of a substance such as a hormone.

perimenopause   A period of time before menopause, sometimes spanning several years, when a woman's menstrual cycles may become irregular and her hormone levels begin to decline. Perimenopause may also extend into the first few years after the menstrual cycle has stopped. Symptoms associated with perimenopause can include changes in cholesterol level, disturbed sleep patterns, hot flashes, and bone loss.

pharmacokinetics   The characteristic interactions of a drug and the body in terms of the drug's absorption, distribution, metabolism, and excretion.

pheromone   A chemical substance secreted by the body that stimulates one or more behavioral responses from other individuals of the same species.

phytoestrogens   Compounds found in plants that are very similar to human estrogens and that may bind with estrogen receptors.

phytohormones   Hormones found in plants.

picogram   One-trillionth of a gram.

pineal gland   A pea-sized organ situated in the brain that secretes melatonin.

pituitary gland   A small, oval endocrine organ attached to the brain that controls growth and development by secreting hormones that regulate and control other endocrine organs.

plaque   In the arteries, a lesion usually made of fats (cholesterol in particular), starches, and calcium that forms under the inner lining of blood vessels and can lead to clogging of the vessels. This process is known as *atherosclerosis.*

plasma   The fluid portion of the blood. It contains soluble components, including clotting factors such as fibrinogen.

PMS   A constellation of symptoms that directly precedes menstruation. These symptoms vary from woman to woman and can include mood swings, instability, irritability, insomnia, fatigue, anxiety, depression, headache, edema, and abdominal pain. PMS stands for *premenstrual syndrome.*

polycystic ovary syndrome (PCO)   An endocrine disorder marked by enlarged cystic ovaries caused by the overproduction of androgens. Symptoms include absence of ovulation, excessive hair growth, amenorrhea, obesity, and infertility.

postmenopause   Those years following the complete cessation of menstruation.

precursor   A substance, cell, or cellular component from which another substance, cell, or cellular component is formed by natural processes. An example is the formation of DHEA from the hormone pregnenolone (pregnenolone is the precursor of DHEA).

pregnenolone   A corticosteroid hormone derived from cholesterol that is the precursor of sex steroid hormones.

premenopause   The time or period of regular menstrual cycling.

premenstrual syndrome   *See* PMS.

progesterone   A sex steroid hormone secreted by the ovary that prepares the endometrium for the implantation of a fertilized egg. Also produced by the placenta during pregnancy to prevent rejection of the developing embryo or fetus.

progestins   A class of hormones that includes natural progesterone and synthetic progestin.

receptor   *See* Hormone receptor.

receptor blocker   A compound that will bind with (engage) a cell receptor but block the action that the receptor would normally provoke. An example is the drug tamoxifen, which engages estrogen receptors but may not set off the normal chain of estrogen events.

SERMs   A classification of drugs that are used as alternatives to the classical estrogens and are designed to target only certain estrogen responses and not others. An example is raloxifene (Evista). SERM stands for *selective estrogen receptor modulator.*

serotonin   A neurotransmitter that affects mood and acts to constrict blood vessels and inhibit gastric secretions.

serum   The clear fluid portion of blood that remains after blood cells, fibrinogen, and fibrin have been removed.

sex hormone binding globulin (SHBG)   A blood protein synthesized in the liver that binds tightly to sex steroid hormones and prevents them from binding with hormone receptors.

sex steroid hormone   Any of a group of hormones produced by the testes, ovaries, and adrenal glands that affect the growth or functioning of the reproductive organs and/or the development of secondary sex characteristics and that have the characteristic ring structure of a steroid hormone. Examples include estrogen, progesterone, DHEA, and testosterone.

steroid hormones   Hormones that are formed in the body from cholesterol and whose molecules have a characteristic ring structure.

stress urinary incontinence   Leakage of urine as a result of coughing, straining, or some sudden voluntary movement due to weakness of the bladder that can occur around the time of menopause.

sublingual   Administered under the tongue in tablets or drops.

synapse   The place at which a nerve impulse passes from one neuron to another.

syndrome   A group of signs and symptoms that occur together and characterize a particular abnormality.

synergy   The interaction of substances in such a way as to create an effect that is greater than the individual effect of each substance.

synthetic hormone   A hormone whose molecules have been manipulated chemically into a patentable molecular structure not identical to the structure of the body's own hormones.

testes   Male reproductive glands that are located in the cavity of the scrotum and produce testosterone and sperm.

testosterone   A hormone produced by the testes and, to a lesser extent, the ovaries and adrenal glands. It is mainly responsible for libido and for inducing and maintaining male secondary sex characteristics.

thymus   An organ located at the base of the neck that produces immune T-cells and is active through puberty.

thyroid   A butterfly-shaped endocrine gland located at the base of the neck that regulates metabolism and produces the hormones thyroxine and calcitonin.

thyroid-stimulating hormone (TSH)   A hormone produced by the brain that governs the release of thyroid hormones from the thyroid gland.

timed release   Term used to describe a medication or other preparation that releases its active ingredients in small amounts over time. Usually refers to a medication that dissolves gradually in the gastrointestinal tract.

transdermal   Delivered through the skin.

triglyceride   A specific kind of body fat. Triglycerides circulate in the blood in the form of lipoproteins. High triglyceride levels are associated with cardiovascular disease.

tubal ligation   A surgical procedure to cut or tie off the fallopian tubes. This prevents ova (eggs) from traveling from the ovaries to the uterus and is used as a method of female sterilization.

up-regulating   Increasing the number of active hormone receptors.

urethra   The canal that carries urine from the bladder to the exterior of the body.

uterine fibroid   A benign (noncancerous) growth in the uterus composed of muscle and fibrous tissue.

uterus   The female organ, also known as the *womb*, that holds and nourishes the fetus during its development. It is composed of a thick outer wall, a layer of smooth muscle, and a mucous lining (the endometrium) containing numerous glands.

vagina   The canal that leads from the uterus to the vulva.

vasomotor   Relating to nerves or nerve centers that supply the muscle fibers of blood-vessel walls and that regulate the amount of blood passing to a particular body part or organ.

vulva   The external parts of the female genital organs.

wild yam   A root vegetable that contains diosgenin, a plant steroid that can be converted in the laboratory to natural, identical-to-human hormones such as estradiol and progesterone.

Bibliography for Further Reading

Ballweg, Mary Lou. *The Endometriosis Source Book*. New York: McGraw-Hill/Contemporary Books, 1995.

Brown, Ellen H., and Lynne P. Walker. *Breezing Through the Change: Managing Menopause Naturally*. Berkeley, CA: Frog Ltd., 1994.

Brown, Ellen H., and Lynne P. Walker. *Menopause and Estrogen: Natural Alternatives to Hormone Replacement Therapy*. Berkeley, CA: Frog Ltd., 1994.

Cabot, Sandra. *Smart Medicine for Menopause: Hormone Replacement Therapy and Its Natural Alternatives*. Garden City Park, NY: Avery Publishing Group, 1995.

Cherniske, Stephen A. *The DHEA Breakthrough*. New York: Ballantine, 1996.

Cloutier-Steele, Lise. *Misinformed Consent: Women's Stories About Unnecessary Hysterectomies*. Chester, NJ: Next Decade, Inc., 2003.

Colgan, Michael. *Hormonal Health, Nutritional and Hormonal Strategies for Emotional Well-Being and Intellectual Longevity*. Vancouver, BC: Apple Publishing, 1996.

Conrad, Christine. *A Woman's Guide to Natural Hormones*. New York: Perigee, 2000.

Corio, Laura E., M.D., and Linda G. Kahn. *The Change Before the Change: Everything You Need to Know to Stay Healthy in the Decade Before Menopause*. New York: Bantam Doubleday Dell, 2002.

Crenshaw, Theresa L. *The Alchemy of Love and Lust: Discovering Our Sex Hormones and How They Determine Who We Love, When We Love, and How Often We Love*. New York: G.P. Putnam's Sons, 1996.

DeGraff Bender, Stephanie, and Kathleen Kelleher. *PMS: Women Tell Women How to Control Premenstrual Syndrome.* Oakland, CA: New Harbinger Publications, 1996.

DeGraff Bender, Stephanie, and Treacy Colbert. *The Power of Perimenopause: A Woman's Guide to Physical and Emotional Health During the Transitional Decade.* New York: Random House, 1998.

Ford, Gillian. *Listening to Your Hormones.* New York: Prima Publishing, 1996.

Golan, Ralph, M.D. *Optimal Wellness.* New York: Ballantine Books, 1995.

Jacobowitz, Ruth S. *150 Most-Asked Questions About Menopause.* New York: Hearst Books, 1993.

Jacobowitz, Ruth S. *150 Most-Asked Questions About Midlife Sex, Love and Intimacy.* New York: Hearst Books, 1995.

Jacobowitz, Ruth S. *150 Most-Asked Questions About Osteoporosis.* New York: Hearst Books, 1993.

Jones, Susan Smith, Ph.D. *A Fresh Start: Accelerate Fat Loss and Restore Youthful Vitality.* Berkeley, CA: Celestial Arts, 2002.

Kelly, Patricia T., Ph.D. *Assess Your True Risk of Breast Cancer.* New York: Henry Holt & Company, LLC/Owl Books, 2000.

Klatz, Ronald, and Robert Goldman. *Stopping the Clock.* New Canaan, CT: Keats Publishing, 1996.

Lark, Susan M., M.D. *The Estrogen Decision.* Berkeley, CA: Celestial Arts, 1996.

Laux, Marcus, and Christine Conrad. *Natural Woman, Natural Menopause.* New York: HarperCollins, 1997.

Lee, John R., and Virginia Hopkins. *What Your Doctor May Not Tell You About Menopause: The Breakthrough Book on Natural Progesterone.* New York: Warner Books, 1996.

Legato, Marianne. *Eve's Rib: The New Science of Gender-Specific Medicine and How It Can Save Your Life.* New York: Harmony Books, 2002.

Legato, Marianne, M.D., and Carol Colman. *The Female Heart.* New York: HarperCollins, 1999.

Legato, Marianne, M.D., and Carol Colman. *What Women Need to Know: From Headaches to Heart Disease and Everything in Between.* New York: Simon & Schuster, 1997.

Love, Susan, M.D. *Dr. Susan Love's Hormone Book: Making Informed Decisions About Menopause.* New York: Random House, 1997.

Nachtigall, Lila, and Joan Rattner Heilman. *Estrogen: The Facts Can Change Your Life.* New York: Harper Perennial, 1995.

Northrup, Christiane, M.D. *The Wisdom of Menopause.* New York: Bantam Doubleday Dell, 2003.

Northrup, Christiane, M.D. *Women's Bodies, Women's Wisdom: Creating Physical and Emotional Health and Healing.* New York: Bantam Doubleday Dell, 2002.

Notelovitz, Morris, and Diana Tonnessen. *Estrogen: Yes or No?* New York: St. Martin's Paperbacks, 1993.

Notelovitz, Morris, and Diana Tonnessen. *Menopause and Midlife Health.* New York: St. Martin's Press, 1993.

Pierpaoli, Walter, and William Regelson, with Carol Colman. *The Melatonin Miracle.* New York: Simon & Schuster, 1995.

Rako, Susan. *The Hormone of Desire: The Truth About Sexuality, Menopause, and Testosterone.* New York: Harmony Books, 1996.

Redmond, Geoffrey. *The Good News About Women's Hormones.* New York: Warner Books, 1995.

Regelson, William, and Carol Colman. *The Super Hormone Promise: Nature's Antidote to Aging.* New York: Simon & Schuster, 1996.

Sahelian, Ray. *Pregnenolone: Nature's Feel-Good Hormone.* Garden City Park, NY: Avery Publishing Group, 1997.

Sahelian, Ray. *DHEA: A Practical Guide.* Garden City Park, NY: Avery Publishing Group, 1996.

Sahelian, Ray. *Melatonin: Nature's Sleeping Pill.* Marina del Rey, CA: Be Happier Press, 1995.

Sapolsky, Robert M. *The Trouble with Testosterone.* New York: Simon & Schuster, 1998.

Sapolsky, Robert M. *Why Zebras Don't Get Ulcers.* New York: W.H. Freeman & Company, 1994.

Shippen, Eugene, and William Fryer. *The Testosterone Syndrome.* New York: M. Evans & Company, 1998.

Sinatra, Stephen, M.D. *Heart Sense for a Woman: Your Plan for Natural Prevention and Treatment.* New York: Plume, 2001.

Vliet, Elizabeth Lee. *Screaming To Be Heard: Hormonal Connections Women Suspect . . . and Doctors Ignore.* New York: M. Evans & Company, 1995.

Weed, Susun S. *Menopausal Years, The Wise Woman Way.* Woodstock, NY: Ash Tree Publishing, 1992.

Wright, Jonathan V., and John Morgenthaler. *Natural Hormone Replacement, for Women Over 45.* Petaluma, CA: Smart Publications, 1997.

Your Own Individualized Natural Hormone Replacement Program

Madison Pharmacy Associates (MPA) was the first pharmacy in the United Sates to compound and individualize natural hormone replacement prescriptions. MPA pharmacists work with physicians and health-care practitioners to customize prescriptions that meet patients' individual hormonal needs.

Your doctor can also get you started in a comprehensive, individualized hormone replacement program. This program will enable you to maintain your hormone levels at well-balanced, beneficial, even youthful levels that are just right for you. It combines the expertise of Aeron LifeCycles Clinical Laboratory and Madison Pharmacy Associates, who pioneered individualized natural hormone replacement, and provides you with the collection supplies for a saliva hormone test and a deoxypyridinoline (Dpd) bone-resorption test. Once you have collected your saliva and urine samples at home, you send them to Aeron LifeCycles for processing. Your results will be sent to you and to your doctor. They can also be sent to Madison Pharmacy Associates, where a clinical counselor will then work with you and your doctor to ensure that you have a hormone replacement program designed to meet your specific needs. After you have begun your program, follow-up tests will be sent to you in order to monitor the effectiveness of your treatment.

To have an information packet sent to you, you can contact either Madison Pharmacy Associates, Inc., or Aeron LifeCycles Clinical Laboratory at the addresses listed on the following page.

Madison Pharmacy Associates, Inc.
Women's Health America, Inc.
1289 Deming Way
P.O. Box 259690
Madison, WI 53725
Toll-free telephone: 800-558-7046
Fax: 888-898-7412
www.womenshealth.com

Aeron LifeCycles Clinical Laboratory
1933 Davis Street, Suite 310
San Leandro, CA 94577
Toll-free telephone: 800-631-7900 (select option 6)
Fax: 510-729-0383
www.aeron.com

Saliva Hormone Testing and Urine Bone-Loss Testing

Saliva hormone testing and urine deoxypyridinoline (Dpd) bone-resorption tests are available from Aeron LifeCycles Clinical Laboratory. Aeron will provide you with the collection supplies necessary for testing your estradiol, estriol, estrone, progesterone, testosterone, DHT, DHEA, and cortisol levels, and your rate of bone loss. Once you have collected your samples of saliva and urine at home and have sent them to the lab for processing, your results can be sent to you and your doctor.

For more information about saliva hormone testing, contact:

Aeron LifeCycles Clinical Laboratory
1933 Davis Street, Suite 310
San Leandro, CA 94577
Toll-free telephone: 800-631-7900 (select option 6)
Fax: 510-729-0383
www.aeron.com

Index